Reducing Stress Fracture in Physically Active Military Women

Subcommittee on Body Composition, Nutrition, and Health of Military Women

Committee on Military Nutrition Research

Food and Nutrition Board

INSTITUTE OF MEDICINE

IOM

NATIONAL ACADEMY PRESS
Washington, D.C. 1998

NATIONAL ACADEMY PRESS • 2101 Constitution Avenue, N.W. • Washington, DC 20418

NOTICE: The project that is the subject of this report was approved by the Governing Board of the National Research Council, whose members are drawn from the councils of the National Academy of Sciences, the National Academy of Engineering, and the Institute of Medicine. The members of the committee responsible for the report were chosen for their special competences and with regard for appropriate balance.

The Institute of Medicine was established in 1970 by the National Academy of Sciences to enlist distinguished members of the appropriate professions in the examination of policy matters pertaining to the health of the public. In this, the Institute acts under both the Academy's 1863 congressional charter responsibility to be an adviser to the federal government and its own initiative in identifying issues of medical care, research, and education. Dr. Kenneth I. Shine is president of the Institute of Medicine.

Support for this project was provided by the U.S. Army Medical Research and Materiel Command through contract no. DAMD17-95-1-5037. The views presented in this publication are those of the Subcommittee on Body Composition, Nutrition, and Health of Military Women and are not necessarily those of the sponsor.

Library of Congress Catalog Card No. 98-87880

International Standard Book Number 0-309-06091-5

Additional copies of this report are available from:

National Academy Press
2101 Constitution Avenue, N.W.
Lock Box 285
Washington, DC 20055

Call (800) 624-6242 or (202) 334-3313 (in the Washington metropolitan area), or visit the NAP's on-line bookstore at *http://www.nap.edu.*

For more information about the Institute of Medicine and the Food and Nutrition Board, visit the IOM and FNB home pages at *http://www2.nas.edu/iom/* and *http://www2.nas.edu/fnb/*.

Printed in the United States of America

The serpent has been a symbol of long life, healing, and knowledge among almost all cultures and religions since the beginning of recorded history. The image adopted as a logotype by the Institute of Medicine is based on a relief carving from ancient Greece, now held by the Staatliche Museen in Berlin.

SUBCOMMITTEE ON BODY COMPOSITION, NUTRITION, AND HEALTH OF MILITARY WOMEN

BARBARA O. SCHNEEMAN (*Chair*), College of Agricultural and Environmental Sciences, University of California, Davis

ROBERT O. NESHEIM (*Vice Chair*), Salinas, California

JOHN P. BILEZIKIAN, Department of Medicine, College of Physicians and Surgeons, Columbia University, New York, New York

NANCY F. BUTTE, Children's Nutrition Research Center, Baylor College of Medicine, Houston, Texas

STEVEN B. HEYMSFIELD, Human Body Composition Laboratory, Weight Control Unit, and Obesity Research Center, St. Luke's-Roosevelt Hospital Center, New York, New York

ANNE LOOKER, Division of Health Examination Statistics, National Center for Health Statistics, Hyattsville, Maryland

GORDON O. MATHESON, Division of Sports Medicine, Department of Functional Restoration, Stanford University School of Medicine, Stanford, California

BONNY L. SPECKER, The Martin Program in Human Nutrition, South Dakota State University, Brookings

Committee on Military Nutrition Research Liaison

GAIL E. BUTTERFIELD, Nutrition Studies, Palo Alto Veterans Affairs Health Care System and Program in Human Biology, Stanford University, Palo Alto, California

Food and Nutrition Board Liaison

JANET C. KING, U.S. Department of Agriculture Western Human Nutrition Research Center, San Francisco and University of California, Berkeley

Military Liaison Panel

CAROL J. BAKER-FULCO, Military Nutrition and Biochemistry Division, U.S. Army Research Institute of Environmental Medicine, Natick, Massachusetts

LT LESLIE COX, USN, Bureau of Naval Personnel, Washington, D.C.

LTC BETH FOLEY, USA, Health Promotion Policy, Department of the Army, Washington, D.C.

JAMES A. HODGDON, Human Performance Department, Naval Health Research Center, San Diego, California

COL ESTHER MYERS, USAF, Biomedical Science Corps for Dietetics, 89 Medical Group, Andrews AFB, Maryland

CDR JANEE PRZYBYL, USN, National Naval Medical Center, Bethesda, Maryland

MAJ JOANNE M. SPAHN, USAF, Nutritional Medicine Service, 3rd Medical Group/SGSD, Elmendorf AFB, Alaska

MAJ VICKY THOMAS, USA, Office of the Surgeon General, Department of the Army, Falls Church, Virginia

CDR FAYTHE M. WEBER, USN, Medical Service Corps, Bureau Medicine and Surgery, Washington, D.C.

U.S. Army Grant Representative

LTC KARL E. FRIEDL, USA, Army Operational Medicine Research Program, U.S. Army Medical Research and Materiel Command, Fort Detrick, Frederick, Maryland

Staff
REBECCA B. COSTELLO (*through May 22, 1998*), Project Director
MARY I. POOS (*from May 23, 1998*), Project Director
SYDNE J. CARLSON-NEWBERRY, Program Officer
SUSAN M. KNASIAK-RALEY (*through April 3, 1998*), Research Assistant
MELISSA L. VAN DOREN, Project Assistant

COMMITTEE ON MILITARY NUTRITION RESEARCH

ROBERT O. NESHEIM (*Chair*), Salinas, California

WILLIAM R. BEISEL, Department of Molecular Microbiology and Immunology, The Johns Hopkins University School of Hygiene and Public Health, Baltimore, Maryland

GAIL E. BUTTERFIELD, Nutrition Studies, Palo Alto Veterans Affairs Health Care System and Program in Human Biology, Stanford University, Palo Alto, California

WANDA L. CHENOWETH, Department of Food Science and Human Nutrition, Michigan State University, East Lansing

JOHN D. FERNSTROM, Department of Psychiatry, Pharmacology, and Neuroscience, University of Pittsburgh School of Medicine, Pennsylvania

ROBIN B. KANAREK, Department of Psychology, Tufts University, Boston, Massachusetts

ORVILLE A. LEVANDER, Nutrient Requirements and Functions Laboratory, U.S. Department of Agriculture Beltsville Human Nutrition Research Center, Beltsville, Maryland

JOHN E. VANDERVEEN, Office of Plant and Dairy Foods and Beverages, Food and Drug Administration, Washington, D.C.

DOUGLAS W. WILMORE, Department of Surgery, Brigham and Women's Hospital, Boston, Massachusetts

Food and Nutrition Board Liaison

JOHANNA T. DWYER, Frances Stern Nutrition Center, New England Medical Center Hospital and Departments of Medicine and Community Health, Tufts Medical School and School of Nutrition Science and Policy, Boston, Massachusetts

U.S. Army Grant Representative

LTC KARL E. FRIEDL, USA, Army Operational Medicine Research Program, U.S. Army Medical Research and Materiel Command, Fort Detrick, Frederick, Maryland

Staff

REBECCA B. COSTELLO (*through May 22, 1998*), Project Director

MARY I. POOS (*from May 23, 1998*), Project Director

SYDNE J. CARLSON-NEWBERRY, Program Officer

SUSAN M. KNASIAK-RALEY (*through April 3, 1998*), Research Assistant

MELISSA L. VAN DOREN, Project Assistant

---

[*] Member, Institute of Medicine.
[†] Member, National Academy of Sciences.

Preface

HISTORY OF THE SUBCOMMITTEE

The Subcommittee on Body Composition, Nutrition, and Health of Military Women (BCNH subcommittee) was established in 1995 through a grant administered by the U.S. Army Medical Research and Materiel Command as part of the Defense Women's Health Research Program. Under the guidance of the Committee on Military Nutrition Research (CMNR), the BCNH subcommittee was asked to evaluate whether existing body composition and physical appearance standards for women in the military conflicted with body composition requirements for task performance and if these same standards might interfere with readiness by encouraging chronic dieting, inadequate intake, and sporadic fitness. The BCNH subcommittee conducted an extensive review of this topic, including a workshop held in September 1996 to gather information on current knowledge and activities relating to achieving fitness and readiness for military women. Additionally, the subcommittee sought to identify factors that would interfere with the readiness and long-term health of military women. A report of this activity has been completed recently (IOM, 1998).

COMMITTEE TASKS AND PROCEDURES

One of the tasks specifically delineated for the BCNH subcommittee was to identify and provide recommendations regarding special nutritional considerations of active-duty military women. An area identified for further study in military women concerns the effect of calcium status, as well as total energy intake, on the incidence of stress fractures in the short term, and osteoporosis in the long term, and the nutrient implications of these conditions. The incidence of stress fractures during basic training is substantially higher in female than in male recruits (IOM, 1992, 1998). This injury has a marked impact on the health of service personnel and imposes a significant financial burden by delaying the training of new recruits. Stress fractures increase the length of training time, program costs, and time to military readiness. In addition, stress fractures and short-term risks to bone health may share their etiology with the long-term risk of osteoporosis.

The incidence of stress fracture in male military recruits has been reported to range from 0.2 percent in U.S. Navy recruits to 4.5 percent in U.S. Marine Corps recruits (Shaffer, 1997). The incidence among females in these same training programs is higher, ranging from 0.7 percent in the Navy to 9.6 percent in Marine officer candidates. The cost incurred due to stress fractures among 2,000 female Marine recruits is estimated to be $1,850,000 annually with 4,120 lost training days resulting in an extended training period for these women. Thus, it could be projected that the costs to the U.S. Army, a service that trains a greater number of recruits annually, would be substantially higher.

Coincidental with the increase in stress fracture incidence was the BCNH subcommittee's concern regarding its possible relationship to the long-term risk of osteoporosis. Because of this higher incidence of stress fractures in female recruits and the resulting increase in length of training time, operating costs, time to military readiness, and the possibility of a shared etiology (or pathogenesis) between short-term (stress fractures) and long-term (osteoporosis) risks to bone health, the DoD, specifically the Headquarters, U.S. Army Medical Research and Materiel Command, requested the BCNH subcommittee to examine this issue and address the following five questions:

1. Why is the incidence of stress fractures in military basic training greater for women than for men?
2. What is the relationship of genetics and body composition to bone density and the incidence of stress fractures in women?
3. What are the effects of diet, physical activity, contraceptive use, and other lifestyle factors (smoking and alcohol) on the accrual of peak bone mineral content, incidence of stress fractures, and development of osteoporosis in military women?
4. How do caloric restriction and disordered eating patterns affect hormonal balance and the accrual and maintenance of peak bone mineral content?
5. How can the military best ensure that the dietary intakes of active-duty military women in training and throughout their military careers do not contribute to an increased incidence of stress fractures and osteoporosis?

The subcommittee decided that in order to address these questions adequately in the short timetable of the proposal, a workshop should be held involving experts in the areas of endocrinology, calcium metabolism, bone mineral assessment, sports medicine, and military nutrition to evaluate the effects of diet, genetics, and physical activity on bone mineral and calcium status. In addition, the report would consider the effects of dietary restriction at the levels observed in military women combined with the physical demands of basic training on short-term bone mineral balance (and the immediate risk of stress fracture) and on the long-term risk of osteoporosis.

The BCNH subcommittee believed it was very important to gather as much information as was available from all military services to determine the incidence of stress fractures in women during basic training and the training conditions imposed to assess whether if, among the services, differences in stress fracture incidence would be observed that might be attributed to differences among the training regimens. The subcommittee also believed it was important to evaluate the average level of women's physical fitness at the beginning of training and to evaluate data on nutrient intakes and other lifestyle factors of recruits that were thought to play a role in the pathogenesis of stress fractures. In addition to the military research personnel who presented data to the subcommittee, a liaison group composed of members of the various uniformed services was asked to attend and provide additional information relevant to the topics discussed. Thus, the discussion at the workshop involved experts in various scientific and clinical disciplines, as well as service personnel who dealt with issues of health and physical performance.

Military personnel in basic training are subjected to extensive physical conditioning over a relatively short period of time to bring them to the level of fitness required to meet the minimum standards for graduation from basic and/or advanced training programs. Thus, the subcommittee felt it was appropriate to compare the incidence of training injuries (stress fractures) observed in female, civilian competitive athletes with that in military women, given similar training environments. This comparison was deemed relevant because the incidence of athletic amenorrhea, a condition associated with estrogen deficiency and an increased risk of lower bone mineral content, is increased in competitive female athletes.

The subcommittee discussed a related but longer-term issue: whether the effect of military training and the military lifestyle (weight management to meet specific weight standards) may be a risk factor for osteoporosis in women in later stages of military service or after retirement. Because the new trainees are largely 18 to 25 years old, no incidence of osteoporosis would be expected in this population.

ORGANIZATION OF THE REPORT

The BCNH subcommittee's conclusions and recommendations, emanating from the workshop, as well as its review of the relevant literature, are organized around the responses to the five task questions initially submitted by the military. This brief report constitutes an evaluation of the relevant factors provided to the subcommittee at the workshop and subsequent discussions in executive session and forms the response to the task questions and the basis for the subcommittee's conclusions and recommendations.

Abstracts from the workshop presentations are included in Appendix A of this report and have undergone limited editorial changes, have not been reviewed by the outside group, and represent the views of the individual authors. Because of time constraints, the responses are largely based on data gathered at the workshop, a review of related relevant publications, and the expertise of the subcommittee.

ACKNOWLEDGMENTS

The subcommittee wishes to acknowledge the help of the IOM's President Kenneth I. Shine, the FNB Division Director Allison A. Yates, and the staff of the BCNH: Study Director Rebecca B. Costello, Staff Officer Sydne J. Carlson-Newberry, Research Assistant Susan M. Knasiak-Raley, Project Assistant Melissa L. Van Doren, and Reports and Information Office Director Michael A. Edington and Associate Claudia M. Carl. Additionally, the subcommittee would like to thank editor Judith Grumstrup-Scott, members of the military liaison panel, and the individuals and organizations who provided information and materials.

This report has been reviewed by individuals chosen for their diverse perspectives and technical expertise, in accordance with procedures approved by the NRC's Report Review Committee. The purpose of this independent review is to provide candid and critical comments that will assist the author and the Institute of Medicine in making the published report as sound as possible and to ensure that the report meets institutional standards of objectivity, evidence, and responsiveness to the study charge. The content of the review comments and draft manuscript remain confidential to protect the integrity of the deliberative process. The BCNH subcommittee wishes to thank the following individuals for their participation in the review of this report: Eldon Wayne Askew, Elsworth Buskirk, Mary Jane De Souza, Robert Marcus, Roger McDonald, Alan Rogol, David D. Schnakenberg, and Richard Wood. Although the individuals listed above have provided many constructive comments and suggestions, responsibility for the final content of this report rests solely with the authoring subcommittee and the IOM.

Contents

Reducing Stress Fracture in Physically Active Military Women

Executive Summary

The incidence of stress fractures during U.S. military basic training is significantly higher in female recruits than in male recruits (Duester and Jones, 1997; Shaffer, 1997). This injury has a marked impact on the health of service personnel and imposes a significant financial burden on the military by delaying the training of new recruits. Stress fractures increase the length of training time, program costs, and time to military readiness. In addition, stress fractures, a short-term risk, may share their etiology with the long-term risk of osteoporosis.

CHARGE TO THE COMMITTEE

As part of the Defense Women's Health Research Program, the U.S. Army Medical Research and Materiel Command requested that the Subcommittee on Body Composition, Nutrition, and Health of Military Women (BCNH subcommittee) evaluate the effects of diet, genetics, and physical activity on bone mineral and calcium status in young servicewomen. The BCNH, a subcommittee of the Committee on Military Nutrition Research (CMNR), was asked to consider the effects of dietary restriction at the levels observed in military women, combined with the physical demands of basic training, both on short-term bone mineral status (and the immediate risk of stress fracture) and on the long-term risk of osteoporosis. In so doing, the subcommittee was asked to respond to the following five questions:

1. Why is the incidence of stress fractures in military basic training greater for women than for men?

2. What is the relationship of genetics and body composition to bone density and the incidence of stress fractures in women?

3. What are the effects of diet, physical activity, contraceptive use, and other lifestyle factors (smoking and alcohol) on the accrual of peak bone mineral content, incidence of stress fractures, and development of osteoporosis in military women?

4. How do caloric restriction and disordered eating patterns affect hormonal balance and the accrual and maintenance of peak bone mineral content?

5. How can the military best ensure that the dietary intakes of active-duty military women in training and throughout their military careers do not contribute to an increased incidence of stress fractures and osteoporosis?

METHODS

In considering the questions posed by the military (and as a follow-on activity to the subcommittee's earlier report, Assessing Readiness in Military Women [IOM, 1998]), the subcommittee consulted with a liaison panel comprising military researchers and health care personnel. A workshop was held in December 1997 to bring together additional military personnel in the areas of training, physical fitness, and military nutrition, as well as civilian researchers and practitioners in the areas of physical fitness and performance, endocrinology, bone mineral assessment, and sports medicine. A focused literature review culled from workshop presentations and selected military and civilian research on the pathophysiology and epidemiology of stress fractures is included in this report.

ORGANIZATION OF THE REPORT

This report responds to the five task questions by evaluating the relevant information provided to the subcommittee at the workshop and subsequent deliberations in executive session, which form the basis for the subcommittee's conclusions and recommendations. Chapter 1 reviews the essential concepts of bone health, Chapter 2 reviews the risk factors for stress fracture, and Chapter 3 examines the effects of energy intake, physical activity, and hormonal factors on bone health. In Chapter 4, the subcommittee provides its responses to the task questions; these responses form the basis for the subcommittee's conclusions, recommendations, and suggestions for additional research. The appendixes contain the agenda and speakers' abstracts from the workshop *Reducing Stress Fracture Among Physically Active Young Servicemembers*, which was held on December 10, 1997 (Appendix A); summary tables of the most recent (1985) Military Recommended Dietary Allowances (Appendix B) and the Food and Nutrition Board's 1997 Recommended Intakes summary table for Calcium and Related Nutrients (Appendix C); and biographical sketches of the subcommittee members (Appendix D).

RESPONSE TO TASK QUESTIONS

1. Why is the incidence of stress fractures in military basic training greater for women than for men?

Stress fracture rates among female Army military trainees during basic combat training are more than twice those reported for male (Deuster and Jones, 1997; Jones and Hansen, 1996; MSMR, 1997). This greater incidence appears to be due in part to the initial entry level of fitness of the recruits and specifically the ability of bone to withstand the rapid, large increases in physical loading. The rate of increase in the intensity, frequency, or volume of impact of loading activities in basic training is a risk factor for stress fractures. In addition, increased stride length and variations in specific exercise activities may contribute to the different site distribution of stress fractures in military women compared with military men. When training regimens are equally imposed on men and women, the resultant stress on the less physically fit increases the likelihood of injury.

Conclusions

Low initial fitness of recruits appears to be the principal factor in the development of stress fractures during basic training. A key component of training programs should be to match closely the rate of musculoskeletal adaptation with the participant, in order to avoid interruption of training for cardiovascular and muscular endurance or fitness. In the training program for female soldiers, rapid and excessive increases in exercise habits and abrupt changes in training load may increase the risk of stress fractures of the lower extremities. The subcommittee concludes that muscle mass, strength, and resistance to fatigue with cyclic loading (bone stress created by excessive or rapid incremental skeletal muscle contraction and loading forces) play a critical role in development of stress fracture. To attain an adequate level of fitness, a training program must include a history of sufficient loading and remodeling within bone if stress injuries and fractures are to be prevented during periods of intense training. Proper footwear and appropriate choice of running surfaces also contribute to the prevention of injuries. Currently there may not be sufficient time during basic training to achieve the aerobic fitness level required to avoid musculoskeletal injury.

Recommendations

A more appropriate fitness standard should be achieved by women entering military service either through a structured program prior to their beginning basic training or through an integrated program within basic training. It is recommended that such a program be designed to start women at a lower level of activity and gradually increase their activity as a transition into full-scale basic training. If a prebasic training program is selected, it should utilize training techniques similar to those employed in basic training.

The BCNH subcommittee recommends a program of basic training that encourages and focuses on (1) avoiding training errors by alternating easy and hard days (i.e., substituting low or nonimpact loading for physical routines that lead to cardiopulmonary fitness), (2) gradual building of skeletal muscle mass with selected strength and endurance activities, and (3) identifying specific exercises that may modify the etiology and site distribution of stress fractures among women and provide ones that do not incur an increased risk for developing stress fractures.

2. What is the relationship of genetics and body composition to bone density and the incidence of stress fractures in women?

Genetics is a determinant of peak bone mass, but it is not known what genes are important nor is it known how important they are in the risk assessment profile for stress fractures.

Body mass and composition *per se* influence bone density. Greater body mass is associated with higher levels of bone mineral mass and density.

Stress fractures are associated not only with reduced skeletal muscle mass and its concomitant increased fatigability and lower fitness levels but also with an excessive skeletal muscle mass and its enhanced strength. Bone stress created by excessive or rapid incremental skeletal muscle contraction and loading forces can cause fractures at specific anatomic sites. However, the major problem for military recruits is likely to be insufficient muscle mass.

Conclusions

It is well recognized that the etiology of stress fracture is multifactorial and that lower bone mineral density is only one contributing factor. Genetics and body mass, specifically muscle mass, are also important determinants in the development of stress fractures. Although current technologies (e.g., dual energy x-ray absorptiometry [DXA], peripheral DXA [pDXA], quantitative computed tomography [QCT], peripheral QCT [pQCT], and ultrasound) may be useful for bone density assessment, which has a wide range of normal values, they cannot be used to screen for stress fracture.

Recommendations

Bone measurements should not be used routinely for screening recruits. Problems with the accuracy of bone mineral content measurements (both specificity and sensitivity) make it difficult to predict stress fractures in military women. Moreover, mean bone mineral density measurements among athletes with stress fracture lie within the normal range.

3. What are the effects of diet, physical activity, contraceptive use, and other lifestyle factors (smoking and alcohol) on the accrual of peak bone mineral content, incidence of stress fractures, and development of osteoporosis in military women?

Energy intake should be adequate (2,000–2,800 kcal/d) to maintain weight during moderate and intensive physical fitness training. A diet adequate in calcium, phosphorus, magnesium, and vitamin D (IOM, 1997) and moderate in sodium and protein (NRC, 1989) should optimize bone health in the short term and theoretically should reduce the long-term risk of developing osteoporosis.

Weight-bearing activity determines the shape and mass of bone. Graded increases in physical activity and resultant increases in the level of musculoskeletal fitness are necessary to ensure sufficient time for loading and remodeling within bone to prevent stress injuries and fractures.

The use of oral contraceptives that contain estrogen with or without progestogens is not considered to have long-term detrimental effects and may benefit bone health. Use of long-acting depot preparations of progestational agents, such as Depro-Provera, has been associated with relative estrogen deficiency. Long-term use of gonadotropin-releasing hormone agonists induces a state of estrogen deficiency and has been associated with bone loss. Cigarette smoking may be a long-term risk factor for the development of osteoporosis, whereas excessive alcohol consumption may be a risk factor in the short term for overall injuries. Whether these lifestyle factors are directly related to the development of stress fractures in the short term or are indirectly related through their long term influence on bone density is not known.

Conclusions

Energy intake by military women should be adequate to maintain weight during intense physical fitness training. Training regimens should provide for a gradual increase of load-bearing activities ("ramp-up"). Nutritional modification of diets of incoming recruits cannot effectively prevent stress fractures during the short term of basic training. The use of oral contraceptive agents is not contraindicated. Exogenous estrogen-progestagen hormones may positively affect peak bone mass reached in adulthood, which may be important for future fracture risks in contrast to the use of long-acting progestagens and gonadotropin-releasing hormone agonists.

Recommendations

Implement measures to ensure that energy intakes by military women are consistent and adequate to maintain weight during intense physical fitness training.

Shift emphasis of the program to one of continual physical fitness, which in turn will assist in the maintenance of weight, fat-free mass, and bone mass in all active servicemembers.

The BCNH subcommittee strongly suggests that the Department of Defense (DoD) consider joining with other federal agencies and programs to educate young adults about the importance of physical activity for health and well-being and to identify those individuals who might be at high risk for stress fracture. This role should be consistent with the DoD's need to have a pool of recruits sufficiently fit for military training.

4. How do caloric restriction and disordered eating patterns affect hormonal balance and the accrual and maintenance of peak bone mineral content?

Caloric restriction or disordered eating may lead to a hormonal disruption that is associated with amenorrhea and an associated estrogen deficiency and loss of bone mineral content (IOM, 1998).

Conclusions

Conditions that induce estrogen deficiency from any cause (e.g., training regimen, diet, weight loss) may adversely affect the skeleton. It is likely that the maintenance of body weight is important in preventing the onset of secondary amenorrhea.

Recommendations

In active-duty servicemembers it is recommended that fitness and body composition assessments be performed frequently. At a minimum, body weight and composition should be evaluated more frequently than the current 6 month intervals. This would foster aherence to practices of healthy weight and physcial fitness and decrease high risk, or disordered eating behaviors.

The prevalence and underlying causes of oligomenorrhea and amenorrhea should be assessed in women undergoing basic training and advanced training and on active duty. Young women in the military should be provided with information about the associations among the menstrual cycle, estrogen sufficiency (including use of contraceptives), bone health, and energy restriction.

5. How can the military best ensure that the dietary intakes of active-duty military women in training and throughout their military careers do not contribute to an increased incidence of stress fractures and osteoporosis?

Nutrition education programs are key to providing information and direction on the choice and nutrient content of appropriate foods. It is important that education programs for military women be aimed at their meeting requirements for total energy needs as well as for nutrients supportive of optimal bone health. With consumption of appropriately higher energy intakes matched to meet the demands of physical training and fitness, higher intakes of calcium should be promoted.

Women should strive to maintain a stable body weight within weight-range standards appropriate for their service and should refrain from episodes of repetitive dieting and weight loss so as not to disrupt normal hormonal rhythms (IOM, 1998). Weight within standard may be achieved through proper diet, selection of nutrient-dense foods, and participation in weight-bearing exercise activities. These measures will be beneficial for the reduction of stress fracture risk in the short term, as well as for osteoporosis prevention in the long term.

Conclusions

Many predisposing factors can alter the menstrual cycle. It is likely that maintenance of appropriate body weight is important in preventing the onset of secondary amenorrhea. To ensure adequate nutrient intakes, female military personnel must be educated on how to meet both energy and nutrient needs. This education is required to enable women to choose foods of higher nutrient density and to maintain a fitness program that will allow greater energy intake.

Recommendations

As recommended in its previous report (IOM, 1998), the BCNH subcommittee "reinforces the requirement for adequate energy and nutrient intakes to reflect the needs of the body at a moderate activity level (2,000–2,800 kcal/d) . . . The subcommittee reinforces the recent efforts of the Army to begin providing complete nutritional labeling of all ration components and to include information to enable identification of nutrient-dense components that would help women meet the MRDAs (Military Recommended Dietary Allowances) at their usual energy intake. . . . The subcommittee recommends nutritional labeling of all dining hall menu items and provision of food selection guidelines to women in garrison" (p. 162).

The military should develop aggressive education programs for military women aimed at helping them identify and select appropriate foods and fortified food products to increase the number of women meeting their requirements for these nutrients. If nutrition education and counseling sessions fail to promote increased intakes, the use of calcium-fortified products becomes essential. Calcium supplements should be recommended under appropriate guidance by the military to meet women's special needs.

RECOMMENDATIONS FOR FUTURE RESEARCH BY THE MILITARY

- Research is needed to define the appropriate fitness level that is required to enable a woman to enter and participate in basic training without incurring an increased risk of stress fractures.
- Data on initial fitness levels should be compiled in recruits from all military services by age, gender, and race/ethnicity.
- Further study is needed to determine the types of activities that may predispose women to stress fractures, especially in the pelvic region and upper leg, and steps should be taken to modify their activities in basic training to lower risk.
- Stress fracture incidence statistics should be collected by age, gender, race/ethnicity, and skeletal site, using a gender-independent, standardized definition of stress fracture and a comparable time frame from all military services for both the basic training and posttraining periods.
- Military research efforts should contribute to identifying those factors, such as diet, lifestyle, and ethnicity, that may contribute to achieving peak bone mass, as well as components of military programs that may interfere with this process.
- Efforts should be made, particularly in women, to investigate more fully the now-preliminary linkages between low skeletal muscle mass and stress fracture risk. Investigators should attempt to determine if this relationship is due to a low skeletal muscle mass effect *per se* or an associated factor such as inadequate initial fitness status.
- Research is needed on the effects of implanted or injectable contraceptives, such as Depo-Provera, on bone mineral density and bone strength. Chemical formulation, dosage, and route of administration require further investigation.
- Research is needed that assesses the effect of dietary energy status of military women on the secretion of hormones that affect bone health, particularly in situations of high metabolic stress.

- The military should continue to gather dietary intake data and evidence concerning calcium intakes throughout the soldier's career, as training programs, food choices, and food supply change over time.
- Based on preliminary data from athletes, the potential loss of calcium in sweat due to physical exertion during training and the impact of high levels of activity on calcium requirements needs to be investigated as possible pathophysiological factors in the development of stress fracture.
- More research is needed to evaluate existing technologies for cost-effective assessment of bone mass. These technologies currently include ultrasound, central and peripheral dual-energy x-ray absorptiometry, and central and peripheral quantitative computer tomography. Ultimately, the cost-benefit analysis of all techniques will have to be addressed for specific uses and populations within the military.
- Mechanical models should be developed which link skeletal muscle mass, force/torque, and bone stress in humans, as well as to improve existing in vivo methods of quantifying components of these models.

1

Pathophysiology and Epidemiology of Stress Fractures in Military Women

ESSENTIAL CONCEPTS

A stress fracture is an overuse injury to bone that results from the accumulation of strain damage from repetitive load cycles much lower than the stress required to fracture the bone in a single-load cycle (Brukner and Bennell, 1997). Stress fractures are commonly associated with vigorous exercise, especially that involving repetitive, weight-bearing loads, like running or marching (Jones et al., 1989).

Although the term *stress fracture* implies a break in bone continuity, many injuries labeled as stress fractures are not associated with a fracture line on plain radiography (Jones et al., 1989). The normal reaction of bone to stress is a localized acceleration of bone remodeling that alters the micro-architectural configuration to better withstand the altered loading environment. Ordinarily this remodeling does not result in pathology, but repeated application of unaccustomed stress may increase the number of activated bone remodeling units. Because the resorption precedes the formation by several weeks in the remodeling process, a short-term loss of bone may result, which ranges from mild levels that do not significantly weaken the bone to levels that are sufficiently high to lead to complete bone failure or fracture (Jones et al., 1989). Because this process exists along a continuum, the clinical features also exist along a continuum from mild to severe.

The biologic adaptability of bone to repetitive strain is mediated by cells surrounded by a mineralized connective tissue matrix of collagen fibers and ground substance. Bone cells arise from different cell lines and carry out various functions including matrix formation, mineralization, and resorption. Osteoblasts are derived from local bone marrow mesenchymal cells and are located on all bone surfaces where active bone formation is taking place (Cowin et al., 1991; Marks and Popoff, 1988). Their main function is to synthesize and secrete the organic matrix of bone. Once osteoblasts stop forming bone, they may either decrease their synthetic activity and remain on the surface of the bone where they are known as bone-lining cells, or they may surround themselves with matrix and become osteocytes. Bone-lining cells are elongated and contain fewer organelles than osteoblasts. The main role of these cells is to contract and secrete enzymes that remove the thin layer of osteoid covering the mineralized matrix. This allows osteoclasts to attach to bone and begin resorption (Buckwalter et al., 1996). Osteocytes comprise more than 90 percent of the bone cells in the mature human skeleton. They are connected to adjacent osteocytes, active osteoblasts, and bone lining cells by numerous cytoplasmic projections that travel in channels (canaliculi) through mineralized matrix (Boivin et al., 1990). These interconnections may allow the cells to sense deformation of bone by mechanical loads and to coordinate the remodeling process.

Osteoclasts are derived from extraskeletal, hematopoietic stem cells (Girasole et al., 1992). They are large, motile, multinucleated cells found on bone surfaces that are undergoing resorption. To resorb the bone matrix, osteoclasts bind to the bone surface and create an acidic environment by secreting proteins and enzymes (Peck and Woods, 1988).

The extracellular matrix of bone is comprised of both inorganic and organic components. The inorganic component contributes approximately 65 percent of the wet weight of bone and consists mainly of calcium and phosphate in crystals of hydroxyapatite (Boivin et al., 1990). Other ions within the bone matrix include carbonate, citrate, fluoride, and magnesium and chloride in much smaller quantities. The inorganic matrix of bone performs two essential functions: it serves as an ion reservoir, and it gives bone most of its strength and stiffness (Buckwalter et al., 1995). The organic components, comprising 20 percent of the wet weight of bone, are collagen fibrils and an interfibrillar ground substance composed of as many as 200 noncollagenous proteins including osteocalcin, osteonectin, osteopontin, and various glycoproteins. These organic constituents give bone its flexibility and resilience (Martin, 1991), and the matrix macromolecules appear to contribute to the structure and functional qualities of bone (Meghji, 1992). The majority of the organic matrix is produced by osteoblasts, the most abundant protein being type 1 collagen (Boivin et al., 1990). Collagen molecules are secreted as procollagen into the extracellular space. They are then assembled into fibrils that are arranged such that spaces exist between molecules to accommodate the calcium and phosphate crystals.

HORMONAL REGULATION OF BONE METABOLISM AND REMODELING

The dynamic processes involved in bone metabolism relate to the events associated with bone formation and bone resorption. The extent to which these two processes are in balance determines whether bone mass will be gained (in youth), conserved (in young adults), or lost (in middle-aged and older adults). As noted earlier, the cells involved in bone formation and bone resorption are the osteoblast and the osteoclast, respectively. Bone markers refer to biochemical moieties that result from the secretory products of these cells or from the formation or breakdown of type 1 collagen, the organic substrate upon which mineralization occurs.

A large number of modulators, including hormones, growth factors, and cytokines,[1] interact at the level of the osteoblast, osteoclast, and other cells to regulate bone remodeling (Margolis et al., 1996). Systemic hormones that either regulate calcium balance or affect bone remodeling include parathyroid hormone, calcitonin, vitamin D, estrogen, progesterone, growth hormone (GH), thyroid hormone, glucocorticoids, and androgens.

Paracrine and autocrine factors involved in bone remodeling include IGF and cytokines such as tumor necrosis factor (TNF)-α, transforming growth factor (TGF)-β, and interleukins (IL). The sequence of molecular events in biochemical coupling of bone resorption to bone formation is not well understood but appears to involve the generation of classical messenger molecules, such as cyclic nucleotides and prostaglandins by load-sensing cells (Marcus, 1996).

In general, systemic endocrine modulators activate both resorption and formation of bone, while paracrine/autocrine factors have more specific effects (Rosen, 1997). Some growth factors are bound to the extracellular matrix in latent form prior to release and activation by other elements in the remodeling cascade. Binding proteins (particularly the IGF-binding proteins) and hormone receptors play critical roles in modulating the activity of hormones and growth factors. Thus, "hormonal and paracrine factors orchestrate a remodeling sequence that also requires a skeletal matrix loaded with inactive growth factors" (Rosen, 1997, p. 1194).

HORMONES THAT REGULATE CALCIUM BALANCE

Parathyroid Hormone

Parathyroid hormone (PTH) is an important hormone regulating bone mineral content (Margolis et al., 1996). PTH stimulates the reabsorption of calcium from the glomerular filtrate, enhances calcium resorption from bone, and increases absorption of calcium from the gastrointestinal tract, secondarily through its effect on renal formation of active vitamin D metabolites. Calcium concentration in the extracellular fluid is the major regulator of PTH secretion (stimulation at low calcium concentrations and inhibition at high calcium concentrations). PTH mobilizes calcium from areas of bone in rapid equilibration with the extracellular matrix and also increases the synthesis of bone enzymes that promote bone resorption and remodeling.

Calcitonin

Calcitonin is a hormone, produced by the parafollicular or C-cells of the thyroid gland, whose principal action is the lowering of serum calcium concentration (Aurbach et al., 1992). Its mechanism of action is through inhibition of bone resorption mediated by cyclic adenosine monophosphate (cAMP).

Continued

[1] Cytokines are small peptides that function as intercellular signals and mediators. Cytokines are produced by many different cells throughout the body. Most cytokines have a diverse variety of actions, depending on the cells they stimulate.

HORMONES THAT REGULATE CALCIUM BALANCE *Continued*

Vitamin D

Vitamin D (1,25 dihydroxyvitamin D_3) is a key hormone in the regulation of intestinal calcium absorption; it increases the fractional absorption of calcium and, to a lesser extent, increases the absorption of phosphate and magnesium. Vitamin D also has a direct anabolic effect on bone cells (Aurbach et al., 1992).

HORMONES THAT REGULATE BONE REMODELING

Estrogen

Estrogen appears to be the critical initiator of the pubertal growth spurt in boys and girls. Estrogen acts primarily, but not exclusively, as an antiresorptive agent on bone. Estrogens suppress osteoblast release of cytokines, which recruit osteoclasts for bone resorption. The cytokine IL-6 is upregulated in estrogen deficiency in most, but not all, studies, and may be responsible for enhanced bone resorption (Margolis et al., 1996). Estrogen deficiency is also accompanied by suppression of osteoblast production of fibronectin, a key element of the extracellular matrix that is important in the recruitment, differentiation, and subsequent function of preosteoblasts. Estrogen has pronounced antiresorptive effects and stimulates bone formation.

Progesterone

Considerably less is known regarding the action of progesterone on human bone. Progesterone appears to modulate bone resorption and protect against bone loss (Graham and Clarke, 1997). It has been postulated that progesterone antagonizes glucocorticoid-mediated bone loss through its ability to act as a ligand for the glucocorticoid receptor (Conover, 1996). Progesterone's effects on estrogen receptors are highly tissue specific, and more work is required to understand the interaction between estrogen and progesterone in human bone.

Growth Hormone

The growth-related effects of growth hormone are primarily mediated by insulin-like growth factor (IGF)-1, a member of the insulin-like gene family. Recent studies have shown that growth hormone and IGF-1 have synergistic effects on bone formation. The effects of IGF-1 are described further in the section on paracrine and autocrine factors.

Thyroid Hormone

Thyroid hormones interact with both nuclear and cell membrane receptors in bone and influence responses of bone cells (Stern, 1996). Thyroid hormone stimulates osteoblast activity, but also promotes resorption through activation of cytokine pathways that lead to osteoclast differentiation. Anabolic effects are more apparent in younger animals and children. Catabolic effects become more prominent at increasing doses. Exogenously administered thyroid hormones are known to increase the risk for bone loss. Estrogens and bisphosphonates can diminish thyroid hormone-stimulated bone loss.

Continued

HORMONES THAT REGULATE BONE REMODELING *Continued*

Glucocorticoids

Direct effects of glucocorticoids on bone are apparent (Lukert and Kream, 1996). Glucocorticoid receptors have been identified on osteoblasts. At high concentrations, glucocorticoids decrease protein, RNA, and DNA synthesis in bone cells and inhibit *COL1A1* gene expression, leading to reduced amounts of type I collagen for bone matrix formation. Glucocorticoids induce osteoporosis; with each remodeling cycle, less bone is replaced, resulting in defective bone formation. Glucocorticoids also exert multiple, indirect effects on bone (Lukert and Kream, 1996). They inhibit pituitary secretion of growth hormone (GH) and cause alterations in insulin-like growth factor (IGF)-binding proteins, leading to a fall in the biologic activity of growth factors with a loss of their anabolic effect on bone. Glucocorticoids also inhibit the secretion of gonadotropin, follicle-stimulating hormone/luteinizing hormone, adrenocorticotrophic hormone, estrogen, testosterone, dehydroepiandrosterone, and androstenedione. Glucocorticoids decrease the transport of calcium and phosphorus and increase the secretion and sensitivity to parathyroid hormone.

Cortisol secreted by the adrenal gland in physiologic amounts is essential for differentiation and function of osteoblasts and osteoclasts (Lukert and Kream, 1996). However, supraphysiologic doses of cortisol inhibit bone formation, thus leading to net bone loss.

Androgens

Administration of androgens (testosterone and 5-α-dihydrotestosterone, dehydroepiandrosterone [DHEA], DHEA-sulfate) exerts positive effects on bone mass either directly or indirectly through increased fat-free mass, reduced renal excretion of calcium, or increased calcium absorption (Schmidt et al., 1996). Evidence from animal models suggests that anabolic steroids act independently of estrogens to increase bone mass and strength. Androgens act through a nuclear androgen receptor, expressed in osteoblast cells.

PARACRINE AND AUTOCRINE FACTORS INVOLVED IN BONE REMODELING

Insulin-Like Growth Factors

Insulin-like growth factors (IGFs) play a key role in bone remodeling by facilitating recruitment of osteoblasts and osteoclasts. IGF-1 is produced in the liver in response to growth hormone (GH) and circulates in combination with IGF-2 and IGF-binding proteins. IGFs are also produced by the osteoblast and stored in latent form in the extracellular matrix. In fact, IGF-2 is the most abundant growth factor stored in human extracellular matrix (Conover, 1996). Other growth factors include transforming growth factor (TGF)-β, basic fibroblast growth factor, and platelet-derived growth factor, all of which can influence production of IGFs by osteoblast cells. While IGFs have some mitogenic effects, their primary action appears to be promotion of osteoblast activity. IGF-1 also stimulates osteoclast recruitment and inhibits collagenase activity (Rosen, 1997). Both IGF-1 and TGF-β are increased with mechanical loading.

Most studies have demonstrated that subcutaneous administration of IGF-1 to animals stimulates linear growth and new bone formation (Rosen, 1997). Short-term treatment of postmenopausal women with IGF-1 results in increased bone turnover. Low-dose IGF-1 (15 μg/kg twice daily) has been shown to increase circulating levels of the markers of bone synthesis, without increasing the markers of bone resorption (Ghiron et al., 1995). No clinical trials with IGF-1 have been conducted in which bone density, fractures, or long-term safety with respect to apoptosis or neoplasms were the primary study outcomes. Further research is needed to establish the role of IGF-1 in treatment of low bone mass or fractures.

Continued

Insulin-Like Growth Factors *Continued*

The presence of estrogen stimulates GH secretion and potentiates the anabolic effect of GH by upregulating GH-receptors on the osteoblast (Slootweg et al., 1997). IGF-1 production is stimulated by estrogen in bone cell cultures and changes the IGF-binding proteins to increase the effective concentration of IGF-1 (Schmidt et al., 1996; Slootweg et al., 1997). Estrogen has also been reported to stimulate TGF-β, another anabolic agent in bone, and may increase extracellular matrix-bound growth factors (Margolis et al., 1996).

Prostaglandins

Cytokines, growth factors, and hormones, as well as mechanical loading, increase prostaglandin production in bone (Pilbeam et al., 1996). A recently identified enzyme, prostaglandin G/H synthase (PGHS-2), apparently mediates much of the prostaglandin production induced with bone remodeling. PGHS-2 is usually expressed at low levels but can be rapidly and transiently induced to very high levels by a number of factors including mechanical loading, interleukin (IL)-1, tumor necrosis factor (TNF)-α, and TGF-β. Prostaglandin production is also increased in bone by endothelial growth factor, platelet-derived growth factor, parathyroid hormone (PTH), and PTH-related protein, and to a lesser extent by vitamin D and thyroid hormone. Nonsteroidal anti-inflammatory drugs (NSAIDs), which inhibit prostaglandin synthesis, suppress new bone formation normally induced by mechanical loading (Pilbeam et al., 1996). Paradoxically, bone resorption induced by immobilization is also blunted by indomethacin or other NSAIDs.

PATHOPHYSIOLOGY OF STRESS FRACTURES

Bone Loading

During physical activity, forces from ground impact and muscle contraction result in bone *stress*, defined as the load or force per unit area that develops on a plane surface, and bone *strain*, defined as the deformation or change in bone dimension. In clinical terms, stress is a measure of the load applied, and strain is a measure of the degree of lengthening or deformation that results. Repetitive strains are essential for the maintenance of normal bone mass. This fact is evident during situations of disuse, immobilization, and weightlessness where dramatic bone loss occurs. Physical activity can lead to increased bone mass as bone adapts to the additional loads placed upon it. However, bone can also lose strength as a result of repetitive loads imposed during normal daily activity if they are applied at too-frequent intervals (Martin and Burr, 1989). This loss of strength is attributed to the formation and propagation of microscopic cracks within bone. If the load is continually applied, these "microcracks" can spread and coalesce into "macrocracks." If repair does not occur, a stress fracture may eventually result.

During physical activity, contact with the ground generates forces within the body. With running, vertical ground reaction force has been shown to vary from 2 to 5 times body weight (Bates et al., 1983; Cavanagh and Lafortune, 1980), and during jumping and landing activities, ground reaction forces can reach 12 times body weight (Deporte and Van Gheluwe, 1989; McNitt-Gray, 1991; Ramey et al., 1985). Transient impulse forces associated with ground reaction forces are propagated upward from the foot, undergoing attenuation as they pass toward the head (Light et al., 1980; Wosk and Voloshin, 1981). A number of factors influence the magnitude, propagation, and attenuation of the impact forces. These include running speed (Frederick and Hagy, 1986; Frederick et al., 1981; Hamill et al., 1983; Nigg et al., 1987), muscular fatigue (Dickinson et al., 1985), type of foot strike (Cavanagh and Lafortune, 1980; Oakley and Pratt, 1988), foot and ankle morphology, body weight (Frederick and Hagy, 1986; Hamill et al., 1983), training surface and terrain (Hamill et al., 1984, Nigg and Segesser, 1988), footwear and lower extremity alignment (Dufek and Bates, 1991).

Accelerated Remodeling

Cyclic loading creates bone stress through intermittent and repetitive skeletal muscle contraction and loading forces. Normal remodeling—the bone's response to cyclic loading due to ground reaction forces—is a sequential process of osteoclastic resorption and osteoblastic new bone formation. This process takes place continuously on both periosteal and endosteal surfaces within cortical bone and on the surface of trabeculae (Parfitt, 1984). The main functions of remodeling are to adapt bone to mechanical loading, to prevent the accumulation of microfractures or fatigue damage (Marcus, 1991; Parfitt, 1988), and to maintain blood calcium levels.

Repetitive loads to bone applied below the load required for single cycle failure (the load that would break bone with a single application) produce cumulative microdamage and initiate the process of accelerated remodeling. Microscopically, the first sign of accelerated remodeling is vascular congestion, thrombosis, and osteoclastic resorption. With continued loading, these signs progress to coalescence of resorbed cavities and then to microfractures with extension to the cortex. For this reason, the clinical response of bone to load can be seen along a continuum from accelerated remodeling to a complete fracture (Figure 1-1). Training influences bone loading and is itself affected by four factors. The volume of training is a function of the total number of strain cycles received by the bone, and the intensity of training (load per unit time, pace, speed) is a function of the frequency of strain cycles applied to bone. The magnitude of each strain and duration of each strain cycle are functions of body weight, muscular shock absorption capability, and lower extremity biomechanical alignment. Impact attenuation is both intrinsic (muscular factors) and extrinsic (equipment and training surfaces). Eccentric muscular strength is important, but even more important is the muscle's ability to resist fatigue; to continue to contract effectively for a sustained period of time. This important factor is a function of metabolic adaptations that occur with training. Foot type and lower extremity biomechanical alignment may affect gait mechanics but altered gait may also occur from fatigue, disease, and injury. Finally, bone health is a major factor that determines the response of bone to loading and is affected by diet and nutrition, genetics, endocrine and hormonal status, the amount of regular exercise, and the presence of bone disease.

Symptamology, physical examination findings, and the results of radiographic imaging studies will be a function of the degree of progression of the injury along the continuum. Initially, accelerated remodeling does not produce symptoms, and plain radiographs will be normal, although magnetic resonance imaging (MRI) may show marrow edema and the nuclear bone scan will show focal uptake of technetium in proportion to the rate of osteoclastic activity. As accelerated remodeling progresses, mild pain will occur some time after the onset of exercise and, with further progression, occur earlier in the exercise bout. Without cessation of loading, pain intensity will increase and will be present even after the exercise bout and with normal activities of daily living. At this point, a technetium bone scan will be positive in all three phases, MRI will show marrow

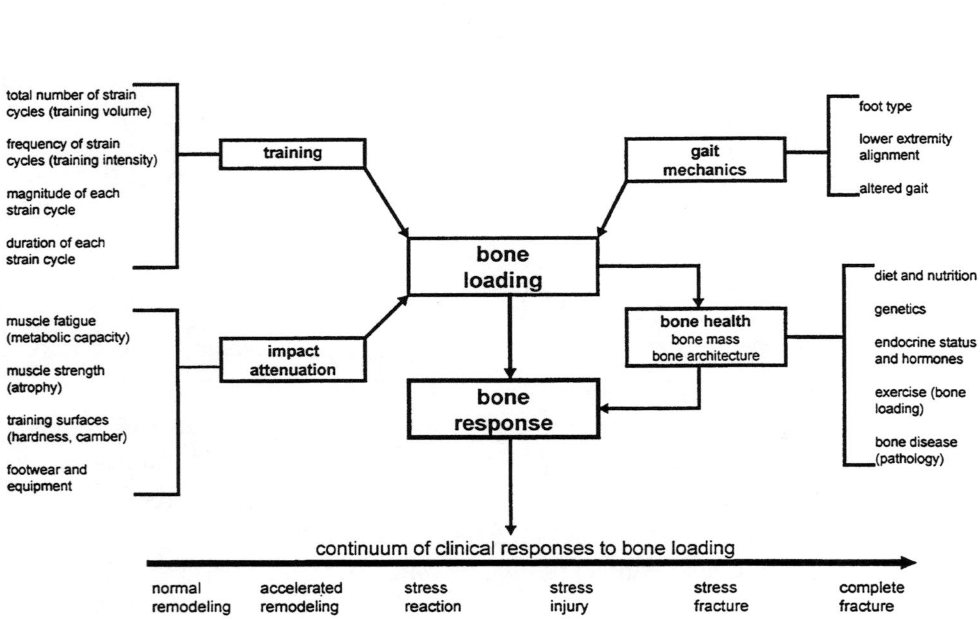

FIGURE 1-1 Determinants of stress fractures. Causal relationships of some of the factors that influence bone health and bone response to loading.

edema, but plain radiographs that specifically detect new bone formation or complete fractures, will still be negative. By the time plain radiographs are positive, a full-blown stress fracture is present. It is important to recognize that this process is on a continuum both physiologically and clinically, and that early intervention is associated with more rapid healing.

Microdamage

Whether microdamage precedes or follows bone remodeling is unclear. Mori and Burr (1993) demonstrated a significant increase in new remodeling events after bone microdamage was induced. Remodeling occurred preferentially in fatigue-damaged regions. However, there were still three times more resorption spaces than microcracks, which suggests that factors other than microdamage also initiate remodeling. Conversely, some human studies suggest that microdamage occurs at pre-existing sites of accelerated remodeling where osteoclastic resorption weakens an area of bone and subjects it to higher strains prior to the addition of new bone by osteoblasts (Burrows, 1956; Engh et al., 1970; Johnell et al., 1982; Johnson et al., 1963; Jones et al., 1989; Michael and Holder, 1985; Roberts and Vogt, 1939; Straus, 1932; Sweet and Allman, 1971). In a temporal series of stress fracture biopsies mainly from the upper tibial cortex in humans, initial histology revealed accelerated cortical resorption (Jones et al., 1989; Johnson et al., 1963). Although no microfracture was seen at this stage, a thin crack was evident in many of the specimens a week later, followed by osteoblastic activity and new bone formation. The study by Li et al. (1985)

employed an exercising rabbit model to assess sequential pathologic changes in the internal structure of the tibia caused by controlled excessive physical activity during a 10-wk period. It was not until the second week that small cracks appeared in the haversian system (the basic unit of structure of compact bone). At this stage, there was obvious osteoclastic resorption and a large number of cavity formations together with increasing subperiosteal osteoblast activity and periosteal proliferation. Most tibiae adapted successfully to changes in bone strain from repetitive loading through internal remodeling, and fractures only appeared if excessive stress continued in a tibia weakened by osteoclastic resorption.

DIAGNOSIS

The diagnosis of stress fracture is based on two factors: (1) local bone pain exacerbated by physical activity and associated with a history of new or recently increased level of physical activity, and (2) plain radiographic abnormalities or focal uptake of technetium on isotopic bone scans at the site of the pain (Matheson et al., 1987a). Computerized tomography and magnetic resonance imaging have also been used to help resolve uncertain cases (Brukner and Bennell, 1997). These techniques vary in their ability to detect the different types of bone pathology associated with a stress reaction. For example, there is often no detectable abnormality on plain x-rays for at least 2 to 3 weeks after symptoms have appeared, and in some cases, abnormalities will never be apparent (Brukner and Bennell, 1997; Matheson et al., 1987b). X-rays have high specificity but poor sensitivity in detecting stress fractures. In contrast, bone scans can detect a developing stress fracture at the stage of increased remodeling, within hours of the injury. Although a bone scan is very sensitive, it will also detect other types of bone lesions, and thus it lacks specificity for the identification of stress fractures. In addition, the bone scan may detect increased bone remodeling that is not associated with any symptoms or immediate danger of bone failure (Matheson et al., 1987a). It is important, then, to correlate results from bone imaging with clinical symptoms when diagnosing stress fractures (Brukner and Bennell, 1997). Different grading systems have been proposed to integrate findings on bone scans and x-rays with clinical symptoms in an effort to promote uniform diagnoses (Jones et al., 1989), but no single system has been adopted. In general, the U.S. military studies reviewed in this report defined stress fractures either through a combination of clinical symptoms and bone image evidence, or a definitive diagnosis noted on the medical record. (Jones et al., 1989).

EPIDEMIOLOGY

Stress fractures were first described in the military as the "march fracture," and in the 1950s stress fractures were identified in the civilian athletic population. In Army recruits undergoing basic training, five injury types are repeatedly cited as accounting for the majority of all training injuries: stress fractures, overuse injuries of the knee, plantar fascitis, achilles tendonitis, and ankle sprains (Jones et al., 1983; Kowal, 1980; Reinker and Ozburne, 1979). Similarly, these same types of injuries are cited as accounting for the majority of all injuries in civilian running and jogging programs (Clement et al., 1981; James et al., 1978; Pagliano, 1980) as well as in training programs for endurance athletes (Fredericson, 1996; Marti, 1988; O'Toole, 1992).

Table 1-1 summarizes the estimated cumulative incidence of stress fractures in U.S. military trainees in several studies conducted over the past 20 years. These estimates vary from 1 to 21 percent in women and from less than 1 to 9 percent in men. The variation in these estimates likely reflects both true and methodological influences. For example, some variation in stress fracture occurrence is to be expected due to differences in training program length and intensity among different military services. However, methodological differences and sampling bias between the studies probably also has an influence. For example, rates reported by Reinker and Ozburne (1979) were based only on subjects who were referred to a specialty clinic. Those reported by Kowal (1980) were based on self-report, and Brudvig and colleagues (1983) used a heterogeneous population (i.e., men and women in both basic and advanced training during a 1-y period) as the denominator when calculating incidence rates in their study. Another factor to consider is the method used to diagnose a stress fracture. For example, focal uptake of technetium on bone scan overestimates the incidence while plain radiography underestimates it. However, the higher occurrence in women than in men appears to be a common finding in military studies, as is a higher occurrence in Caucasians than in non-Caucasians. Stress fracture rates in military servicewomen shown in Table 1-1 are approximately 1.2 to 11 times higher than in men. This gender pattern was also observed in a recent study of Army-wide hospitalizations for spontaneous femur fractures, with female soldiers on active duty having a tenfold higher hospitalization rate than males (MSMR, 1997). Data from Marine recruits suggest that differential symptom reporting may play a role in the observed gender differences in stress fracture, as female recruits are more likely to report overall injury symptoms than males (Shaffer, 1997). Additional data from other services would be useful to support this possibility. The small amount of data by race in Table 1-1 suggest that the fracture rate in Caucasians is 3 to 8 times higher than in African Americans. Hospitalization rates for femur stress fractures were almost twice as high in Caucasian, non-Hispanic soldiers as in African Americans, and almost 30 percent higher than in Hispanics (MSMR, 1997). More data would be useful to confirm the actual magnitude of the African American/Caucasian difference in stress fracture rates.

Most studies on stress fracture occurrence in the military have focused on the basic training period. The small amount of data available suggest that, although injury rates decline after basic training, they are still a problem. For example, nearly 40 percent of the hospitalizations for spontaneous femur fractures in active-duty Army personnel occurred during the third or fourth month of training, which corresponds to the period of advanced individual training (AIT) for most soldiers (MSMR, 1997). Overall injury rates among female Army trainees were lower in advanced training (30%) than in basic combat training (BCT, 52%), and no longer differed from that seen among male trainees (24% during AIT and 27% during BCT) (Knapik and Henderson, 1997). Interestingly, the injury rate during AIT was 43 percent among women who were allowed to attend civilian schooling between BCT and AIT. The study authors speculated that this higher injury rate might be due to loss of physical conditioning in the extended period between basic and advanced training.

Data on stress fracture occurrence among civilians are limited to studies of athletes, and, with few exceptions, these are predominantly case reports or cross-sectional studies that cannot

TABLE 1-1 Estimated Cumulative Incidence of Stress Fractures (%) among U.S. Military Trainees

Study	Sample	Women	Men
Protzman and Griffis, 1977	West Point Cadets	10.0	1.0
Reinker and Ozburne, 1979	Army trainees	12.0	2.0
Kowal, 1980	Army trainees	21.0	4.0
Scully and Besterman, 1982	Army trainees	—	1.3
Brudvig et al., 1983	Army trainees:		
	Total sample	3.4	0.9
	White	11.8	1.1
	Black	1.4	0.2
Gardner et al., 1988	Marine recruits		
	Total sample	—	1.3
	White	—	1.6
	Black	—	0.6
	Hispanic	—	0.7
Pester and Smith, 1992	Army recruits	1.1	0.9
Jones et al., 1993	Army recruits	12.3	2.4
Shaffer et al., 1994	Marine Recruits	—	3.8
Jones, 1996	Army recruits		
	Week 8 of BCT (Company A&B)	6.0	3.8
	Week 7 of BCT (Company C&D)	8.9	3.6
	Week 6 of BCT (Company E&F)	5.1	1.4
Shaffer, 1997	Navy and Marines:		
	Navy Seals	—	8.9
	Marine Corps Recruits:		
	San Diego	—	2.2
	Parris Island	5.1	3.5
	Navy Training	0.6	0.2
	Marine Corps Officer Candidate School	9.8	—
Winfield et al., 1997	Marines	11.5	7.0

NOTE: BCT, basic combat training; —, not determined.
SOURCE: Adapted from Deuster and Jones (1997) and Jones and Hansen (1996).

provide an estimate of true incidence (Brukner, 1997). Estimates of stress fracture incidence in civilian female track and field athletes or runners from two prospective studies were roughly 20 percent (Bennell et al., 1996; Zernicke et al., 1993), while a third prospective study that focused on athletes from various sports reported a 7 percent incidence (Johnson et al., 1994). This variation in rates may reflect both true and methodological differences in these studies. In contrast to findings among military trainees, stress fracture rates among civilian female athletes are more similar (i.e., 1–3.5 times) to those in male civilian athletes (Brukner and Bennell, 1997). However, data for civilian athletes may not be directly comparable with those for military recruits due to differences in training, footwear, and initial fitness level (Bennell et al., 1996; Montgomery et al., 1989).

The skeletal site of the stress fracture may vary between men and women in the military (Table 1-2). The data in Table 1-2, although based on small sample sizes, suggest that female trainees are more likely to develop stress fractures in the upper leg and pelvis, while male trainees are more likely to have lower extremity stress fractures. Pelvic and femur fractures require more time for rehabilitation and may result in more disability and operational costs than stress fractures that occur below the knee. For example, hospitalizations for spontaneous femur fractures in active-duty Army soldiers between 1993 and 1996 resulted in more than a month of lost duty days on average, and more than a total of 7 lost duty years (MSMR, 1997). More than half of the hospitalized cases required surgery for internal fixation of the fracture. Factors causing this variation in site distribution of stress fractures in military women may include alterations in stride length (women are encouraged to march and keep the same stride as men, which is longer than what they are accustomed to) and the form in which they prepare to perform push-ups (women drop to their knees, men to their hands) (Shaffer, 1997). If an altered site distribution is confirmed, these findings further underscore a different pattern of stress fractures in military women, since, besides being more common, they tend to occur in skeletal sites with varying degrees of risk.

Military Training Programs

Military basic training programs vary from a duration of 6 weeks for basic military training (BMT) in the Air Force, to 11 to 13 weeks for Marine Corps recruit depot (MCRD), 9 weeks for Navy recruit training command (RTC), and 8 weeks for Army BCT. Table 1-3 summarizes the key features of each of these service programs.

Army

Most recruits prepare to enter the service and basic training through participation in the Delayed Entry Program (DEP) that exists in most recruiting centers. Between 70 and 80 percent of all recruits across the services spend at least 30 days in this program. Attendance and adoption of physical training recommendations (a minimum of once a month and no more than 90 minutes/exercise session) have been poor (Report of the Federal Advisory Committee on Gender-Integrated Training and Related Issues, to the Secretary of Defense, December 1997). Male DEP participants are required to correctly perform 13 push-ups and females must perform 1 push-up prior to enlistment. Physical training (PT) programs may consist of non-contact team sports (i.e. softball, touch or flag football, volleyball, basketball). Physical conditioning exercises may also be used instead of, or in combination with, those mentioned above. DEP training programs are not designed to replicate basic training conditions and environment, or to push members to meet the

TABLE 1-2 Anatomical Site of Stress Fracture among U.S. Military Trainees

			Percent of All Stress Fractures			
			Women		Men	
Study	Sample	Anatomical Site	*n*	%	*n*	%
Protzman and Griffis, 1977	West Point cadets	Foot	4	40	5	42
		Tibia/fibula	3	30	7	58
		Femur, incl. neck	3	30	0	0
Brudvig et al., 1983	Army trainees	Foot	65	43	94	65
		Tibia/fibula	54	36	34	24
		Femur, incl. neck	17	11	12	8
		Pelvis	15	10	4	3
Iannacchione et al., 1995	Air Force trainees	Ankle/foot	18	58	6	75
		Shin/lower leg	10	32	2	25
		Upper leg	3	10	0	0
Shaffer, 1997	Marine recruits	Foot	*	26	*	46
		Tibia	*	26	*	50
		Femur	*	23	*	2
		Pelvis	*	25	*	2

* Data are not available.

Army physical fitness standards applicable to active duty servicemembers, (USAREC Reg 601-95). Prior to departure for basic training, recruits to a Military Entrance Processing Site (MEPS) where a history and physical exam is performed and a form SF 88-93 is completed. Medical officers evaluate each recruit's physical capabilities based on a thorough medical history and examination. Recruits can be referred for orthopedic consultation if indicated by history or by observation of completion of a set of floor exercises designed to screen for musculoskeletal abnormalities (Sgt. Waters, Baltimore, MD MEPS, Personal communication, 1998).

Within the first couple of days of arrival at Army BCT, recruits will undergo a *prediagnostic* qualifying test. A female recruit must be able to do at least one push-up, and a male recruit must be able to do at least 13 push-ups. If these criteria are not met, the recruit is then referred to the Fitness Training Unit (FTU), which is designed to take the extremely poor performers and work with them through a specially designed training program to assure they can pass the entry criteria for push-ups, sit-ups, and a 2-mi run. Approximately 5 to 8 percent of a recruiting class are referred to the FTU. While assigned to the FTU, the soldier is provided fitness instruction as well as time to work on fitness activities. These fitness activities include aerobic and anaerobic exercises, but push-up performance remains the standard by which a soldier is assessed for advancement to BCT. A trainee has up to 21 days to achieve successfully the push-up standards of the fitness company. As soon as the female recruit can do 6 push-ups and the male recruit 20 push-ups, they re-enter BCT. If recruits are unable to achieve these standards, they are separated from the Army on grounds of not meeting medical fitness standards (Department of the Army, AR 350-15, AR 350-41).

TABLE 1-3 Summary of U.S. Military Training Programs

	Army	Navy	Marine Corps	Air Force
Course duration (includes fitness + academic training)	BCT: 8 wks AIT: varies greatly OSUT*: 13 wks	RTC: 9 wks	MCRD Men: 11 wks Women: 13 wks	BMT: 6 wks
Gender Integrated	Yes: at some sites	Yes	No	Yes
Stratify by fitness level on entry	Yes: if fails pre-diagnostic; assigned to FTU	No	PCP assignment available (pending initial strength test results)	Yes: 5 levels for women, 4 levels for men
Fitness training emphasis	CR endurance (running, marching) Muscular endurance (push-ups, sit-ups)	CR endurance (running, marching) Muscular endurance (push-ups, sit-ups)	CR endurance (running, modified interval training) Muscular endurance (circuit resistance training)	CR endurance (running for time instead of distance) Muscular endurance (circuit resistance training)
Physical fitness testing requirements for graduation	BCT for age group 17–21 by event score† 2-mi run time (min) Men: 16:54 Women: 19:54 Sit-ups (2 min) Men: 42 Women: 40 Push-ups (2 min) Men: 32 Women: 13 AIT and OSUT 2-mi run time (min) Men: 15:54 Women: 18:54 Sit-ups (2 min) Men: 52 Women: 50 Push-ups (2 min) Men: 42 Women: 18	RTC for age group 17–19# 1.5-mi (run/walk) Men: 12:45 Women: 15:00 Curl-ups (2 min) Men: 45 Women: 40 Push-ups (2 min) Men: 38 Women: 18	MCRD for age group 17–26 Sit-ups⊕ (2 min) 45 (min) Dead hang pull-ups (men) 3 (no time limit) Flexed arm hang (women) 15 s 3-mi run time (min) Men: 28 Women: 31	BMT for age group under 30 2-mi run time (min) Men: 18 Women: 21 Sit-ups (within 2 min) Men: 45 Women: 38 Push-ups (within 2 min) Men: 30 Women: 14
Recruits trained yearly (*n*)	Men: 55,496 Women: 13,329	Men: 45,000 Women: 9,000	Men: 45,000 Women: 2,500	34,500
Dropout rate (includes all causes)	12–15% (3% due to physical fitness)		Men: 10–12% Women: 15–18%‡	9.13%§

NOTE: BCT, basic combat training; AIT, advanced individual training; OSUT, one-station unit training; RTC: recruit training command; MCRD, Marine Corps recruit depot; BMT, basic military training; FTU, fitness training unit; PCP, Physical Conditioning Platoon; CR, cardiorespiratory.

* OSUT is a combination of BCT and AIT for some military occupational specialties. † For BCT, must score > 150 event pts (>50 pts each category); for AIT, must score > 160 event pts (> 60 pts each category). Event points stratified by age groups. ‡ Approximately 50% due to medical problems. § Reasons for discharge: total 1,375 recruits discharged during study period (Recruit Fitness Study, 9/95); 731 for new or pre-existing medical reasons; men, 55.6% injury related; women, 46.8% injury related. # Satisfactory score constitutes passing. ⊕ Effective 1 Jul 98, crunch sit-up will replace standard sit-up: 50 (2 min).

SOURCE: *Army*, L. Tomasi (personal communication, U.S. Army Physical Fitness School, Ft. Benning, Ga., 1998); *Navy and Marine Corps*, CDR R. A. Shaffer (personal communication, Naval Health Research Center, San Diego, Calif., 1998) Lt. Col. L. Pappa (personal communication, Training and Education Division, Marine Corps Combat Development Command, Quantico, Va., 1998); *Air Force*, MSGT L. Caramante (personal communication, 939th Training Squadron, Lackland AFB, San Antonio, Tx., 1998.)

At the end of the first week of BCT, a *diagnostic* training test is performed (1- or 2-mi run, sit-ups, and push-ups) as a screening and introductory testing measure. Over the next 6 to 7 weeks, the physical training continues in a regimental fashion. Certain factors are considered in the design of all military fitness training programs. These factors, Frequency, Intensity, Time and Type or "FITT," are the rationale for the Army's fitness program (Table 1-4). At approximately7 weeks, the recruits take a repeat physical fitness test.[2] They must score a minimum of 50 points in each event and a minimum total of 150 points to graduate from BCT and proceed to the AIT course.

When recruits fail, their cases are reviewed to determine reason(s) for failure. Approximately 3 percent leave BCT for physical fitness reasons and approximately another 12 percent leave for medical reasons (for example, cellulitis, stress fractures, pre-existing conditions).

All Army recruits who enter advanced training must have achieved a minimum fitness test score of 150 points. Depending on the training course (infantry, artillery, armor, military police), the duration of time in advanced training may vary. For infantry AIT, the course is 13 weeks. To graduate from advanced training, a recruit must achieve 60 points in each event and a total of 180 points.

Guidance on the planning and development of physical fitness training is outlined in the Army's *Physical Fitness Training* manual (FM 21-20, 1992). The manual provides guidelines for developing programs that will improve and maintain physical fitness levels for all Army personnel and includes specific chapters devoted to physical training during initial entry training and to injuries.

Navy and Marine Corps

In response to concerns about the incidence of musculoskeletal injuries among Marine Corps recruits, the Marine Corps convened several panels of Marine Corps and Navy researchers and sports physicians in 1995. These panels reviewed the Marine Corps Recruitment Depot (MCRD) physical training programs and issued a report that resulted in program revisions and the creation of a user's manual, *A Physical Training Program to Reduce Musculoskeletal Injuries in U.S. Marine Corps Recruits* (Almeida et al., 1997). The revised program was tested in 1995,

---

[2] The physical fitness test (PFT) is used as more of a gauge of physical fitness and a form of competitive review. In order to train recruits and motivate active-duty soldiers to do well on, and maintain a level of fitness, a point system was developed for grading PFTs. A maximum score for each of the three test events, push-ups, sit-ups, and 2-mi run was set at 100 points. A maximum of 300 points can be earned for the three events (push-ups, sit-ups, and 2-mi run). Each gender and age group has its own standards and there are 8 age groups, thus 16 different performance expectations (2 × 8) times 3 events to total 48 different age-gender performance standards. A maximum point score that can be achieved in any of the 48 standard "cells" is 60 points, or 180 total points (FM 21-20, 1992).

TABLE 1-4 FITT Factors Applied to Physical Conditioning Program

Cardiorespiratory Endurance	Muscular Strength	Muscular Endurance	Muscular Strength and Muscular Endurance	Flexibility
Frequency 3–5 times/wk	3 times/wk	3–5 times/wk	3 times/wk	Warm-up and cool-down: Stretch before and after each exercise session Developmental stretching: To improve flexibility, stretch 2–3 times/wk
Intensity 60–90% HRR	3–7 RM	12+ RM	8–12 RM	Tension and slight discomfort, Not pain
Time 20 min or more	The time required to do 3–7 repetitions of each exercise	The time required to do 12+ repetitions of each exercise	The time required to do 8–12 repetitions of each exercise	Warm-up and cool-down stretches: 10–15 sec/stretch Developmental stretching: 30–60 sec/stretch
Type Running Swimming Cross-country skiing Rowing Bicycling Jumping rope Walking/hiking Stair climbing	Free weights Resistance machines Partner-resisted exercises Body-weight exercises (push-ups/sit-ups/pull-ups/dips/etc.)			Stretching: Static Passive PNF

NOTE: FITT, frequency, intensity, time and type; HRR, heart rate reserve; RM, repetition maximum; PNF, proprioceptive neuromuscular facilitation. SOURCE: FM 21-20, 1992.

further modifications were made, and the new program was implemented in 1996 (personal communications, LTC Leon Pappa, Quantico VA, 1998; J. Hodgdon, NHRC San Diego, 1998). The modified training program targeted the average U.S.Marine Corps recruit, who is in poor to fair physical condition on arrival at MCRD. The new program contained a number of features:

• a more progressive ramp-up of the running component in terms of distance, frequency, and intensity;
• fewer formation runs and more individual runs;
• addition of conditioning runs during Second Phase,
• decreased total running mileage and increased total muscle strength and endurance training for a more balanced conditioning program;
• modification of the Daily 7 calisthenics and the circuit course exercises to (a) target all major muscle groups, (b) enhance the strength training stimulus, and (c) reduce injury risk;
• implementation of a comprehensive flexibility training program;
• addition of exercise warm-up and cool-down routines;
• a more progressive ramp-up of load-bearing conditioning hikes; and
• modification of the scheduling of different physical training events to maximize training benefit and minimize the risks of overtraining and overuse injuries.

Through the implementation of the modified physical training program, stress fractures in male Marine Corps recruits have been reduced by 50 percent with no decrease in fitness level at graduation.

Based on the original panel recommendations and the experiences of the Marine Corps with the modified physical training program, the Navy has implemented a similar curriculum modification for female recruits, resulting in a 49 percent decrease in lower extremity overuse injuries.

Air Force

In the spring of 1994, the 737th Training Group at Lackland Air Force Base, the group responsible for BMT, was required to increase the fitness levels of its trainees. The Air Force Office of Prevention and Health Services Assessment (OPHSA) provided the consulting expertise for the design of a new physical conditioning (PC) program. The program included five key features:

• an initial recruit fitness assessment,
• separation into ability groups,
• running for time instead of distance,
• circuit resistance training with sandbags as weights, and
• intertrainee encouragement.

In addition, OPHSA developed student academic material and collaborated on lesson plans for a new 4 h block of class instruction time that focused on exercise physiology and fitness principles. Recommended modifications to the PC program were field tested, and dramatic improvements in the 2-mile run times were noted, as well as larger gains for push-ups and pull-ups in male trainees. Injury rates were not proportionally increased in males, and only a small increase was noted in the proportion of women reporting injuries. However, hip/leg injuries for women and ankle/foot injuries for men remained constant throughout basic training. Results from the field study validated the prototype PC program and demonstrated significant improvements over the existing PC program. Based on these findings, OPSHA recommended adoption of the new program in February 1995.

Fitness Levels of Recruits

Initial fitness levels have been found to be strongly related to subsequent development of stress fractures during basic training (Canham et al., 1996; Deuster and Jones, 1997; Shaffer, 1997). Some investigators have reported that differences in injury incidence no longer exist between genders when men and women of the same aerobic fitness levels are compared (Canham et al., 1996). Also, because women are smaller in body size, their average muscular strength may be less than that of men, but when expressed per pound of body weight, men's and women's strength may be similar (IOM, 1998). Table 1-5 summarizes data on initial fitness levels by gender in Army and Air Force recruits, respectively. Women had lower initial fitness scores than men, except for flexibility (Bell et al., in press; Canham et al., 1996). Data from Canham and colleagues (1996) suggest that fitness levels of all Army recruits have declined slightly over time between the mid- to late-1980s and the mid-1990s. One anecdotal report indicated that 75 percent of the incoming Army recruits who do not meet initial fitness standards are female (Bell, 1988). From experiences in Operation Desert Shield/Storm, it was apparent that many Air Force service personnel were ill-prepared for the rigors of the desert. This was attributed to the lack of preparation achieved in basic training. In female Air Force recruits, run test failures at baseline were reported to be 53 percent compared with 33 percent in male recruits (Jaeger et al., 1996).

The Navy reports that greater than 30 percent of Marine Corps recruits were in poor to very poor condition (i.e., 30 percent of incoming recruits cannot run 1.5 mile in less than 12 minutes) (Shaffer et al., 1994).

By the completion of the 8-wk Army BCT, women still performed fewer push-ups and ran more slowly than men, but women showed greater improvement over initial levels (i.e., improvements in sit-ups, push-ups, and run times were 98, 156, and 23 percent for women compared with 44, 54, and 16 percent for men) (Stoneman, 1997). Thus, it would appear that women are capable of achieving significant improvements in cardiovascular fitness and muscular endurance but may require a longer period to achieve levels comparable to men.

TABLE 1-5 Physical Fitness Levels of Military Recruits Entering Basic Training

Study	Characteristic	Women	Men
U.S. Army training programs			
Bell et al., in press			
Pre-BCT fitness 1988	Maximum handgrip strength (kg)	67.3	117.2
	Flexibility (cm)	32.6	34.8
	Initial 1-mi run time (min)	10.1	7.6
	Initial sit-ups (*n*)	30.9	43.7
	Initial push-ups (*n*)	10.9	32.4
Canham et al., 1996, BCT			
Ft. Jackson 1984	2-mi run time* (min)	20.2	15.6
	Sit-ups (*n*)	40	55
	Push-ups (*n*)	12	31
Ft. Jackson 1988	2-mi run time* (min)	20.3	16.4
	Sit-ups (*n*)	34	44
	Push-ups (*n*)	10	31
Ft. Leonard Wood 1995	2-mi run time* (min)	22.5	17.7
	Sit-ups (*n*)	33	41
	Push-ups (*n*)	11	31
Bell et al., in press			
Post-BCT fitness 1988	End 2-mi run time (min)	17.4	14.0
	End sit-ups (*n*)	61.3	63.0
	End push-ups (*n*)	27.9	49.8
U.S. Air Force training programs†			
Wilborn, 1997		323	423
Baseline	2-mi run time (min)	21:42	17:21
	sit-ups (*n*)/2 min	31	42
	push-ups (*n*)	15	39
Final	2-mi run time* (min)	18:09	14:56
	sit-ups (*n*)/2 min	49	57
	push-ups (*n*)	27	50

NOTE: Basic combat training (BCT) = 8 weeks.
*Predicted from 1-mi run time to allow comparison with physical fitness training scores.
†Random sample data from Basic Military Training Physical Conditioning program trainees at Lackland Air Force Base.

SUMMARY

A stress fracture occurs when changes in physical activity produce a site-specific mechanical "load." This load results in an acute imbalance between the rate of osteoclastic resorption and the rate of osteoblastic new bone formation. Bone metabolism and remodeling are regulated by a large number of modulators including hormones, growth factors, and cytokines that interact at the level of the osteoblast, osteoclast, and other cells to regulate bone remodeling. Systemic hormones that affect bone remodeling include parathyroid hormone, calcitonin, vitamin D, estrogen, progesterone, growthhormone, thyroid hormone, glucocorticoids, and androgens. Stress fractures are diagnosed using a combination of clinical symptoms and results from bone imaging studies.

Estimates of stress fracture rates in military women during basic training range from 1 to 20 percent, while rates in military men range from less than 1 to 9 percent. This variation likely reflects both true variation in rates and methodological differences between the studies. Rates in civilian female athletes show less variation and do not substantiate the theory that a true difference exists. Stress fractures are more common in military women than in men, with estimates in women being 1.2 to 11 times higher than in men in the various studies performed to date. The difference in findings between military trainees and civilian athletes may reflect differences in training, footwear, and initial fitness levels between these two groups. Female military trainees appear to be more likely to suffer stress fractures in the upper leg and pelvis than are males. These fractures are more costly in terms of rehabilitation and potential disability than those that occur in the lower leg. Female military trainees also appear to be more likely to enter training with low fitness levels, which increases their risk of incurring a stress fracture, presumably due to premature muscle fatigue.

2

Bone Health and Risk Factors

The most important modifiable risk factors associated with bone mass are hormonal status, physical activity, and nutrition. Nonmodifiable factors, such as hereditary and familial factors, have a strong influence on bones, especially on the spine and less so on the femoral neck (Kelly and Eisman, 1992; Krall and Dawson-Hughes, 1993; Sambrook et al., 1993). The impact of these risk factors extends throughout an individual's life.

Individuals are thought to attain their peak bone mass in the age range of military recruits, although the timing may vary by skeletal site. For example, peak bone mass in the hip is achieved by age 16 years (Weaver, 1997). In a group of females aged 11 to 32 years, 92 percent of the maximal total-body bone mass observed was present by age 18, and 99 percent was present by age 26 (Teegarden et al., 1995). Bone mass, which may continue to accumulate upto age 30, may be adversely affected by inadequate calcium intakes during adolescence and early adulthood. Achievement of an insufficient peak bone mass is considered one of the major risk factors for subsequent development of osteoporosis (Lu et al., 1994; Recker et al., 1992; Teegarden et al., 1995). Among young adults, skeletal mass is generally greater in males than in females, and greater in blacks than in whites. In addition, bone loss begins at an earlier age in females than in males, and although onset of loss in females begins before menopause, the rate of skeletal loss in some females is distinctly accelareted the first five years after menopause (Dawson-Hughes et al., 1990). Consequently, net skeletal mass is lowest in the menopausal white female, which increases the predisposition to skeletal fracture.

It is unclear whether increasing calcium intake in children and adolescents will have an impact on peak bone density or future risk of fracture. However, it has been demonstrated that increasing calcium intake from food sources (from 900 to 1500 mg daily) prevents bone loss from the spine in premenopausal women (Baran et al., 1990)

BONE MINERAL DENSITY

Peak bone mass is most often measured and referred to as bone mineral density (BMD, g/cm^2)[1] because of the strong correlation between BMD and bone strength (Bouxsein and Marcus, 1994; Moro et al., 1995). Many studies have found associations between low BMD and history of previous fracture (Gluer et al., 1996; Honkanen et al., 1991). However, these studies are difficult to interpret because immobilization and inactivity following a fracture may have contributed to the reduced BMD as noted by several investigators (Henderson et al., 1992; Kannus et al., 1994). Those individuals with a tibial fracture who were immobilized for longer periods (mean of 27 weeks) had a deficiency in bone density at a mean of 9 years following the fracture (Kannus et al., 1994). Thus, it is not clear whether low BMD led to the fracture or resulted from the fracture.

Prospective studies have also found a relationship between increased fracture risk and low BMD (Kelsey et al., 1992). Low bone mineral content (BMC) or BMD as measured by either procedure involving radiation (such as dual energy x-ray absorptiometry [DXA], single photon absorptiometry [SPA], or radiographic absorptiometry) or ultrasound is significantly associated with an increased risk of future fracture in older women as illustrated in a recent meta-analysis (Marshall et al., 1996). The majority of studies of fracture risk and BMC have been completed in older, often postmenopausal, women; few studies have investigated young adults. The number of published reports comparing the relationship of BMD to the incidence of stress fractures is comparatively fewer than for complete fractures. In a 12-mo prospective study, stress fracture occurrence was associated with low BMD in female, but not male, athletes (Bennell et al., 1996). A longitudinal study conducted in 1,319 recruits at the Naval Health Research Center in conjunction with Johns Hopkins University found a lower BMD of the tibia and femur (using DXA) in recruits who sustained stress fractures ($n = 59$) during basic training compared with those recruits without stress fractures (Beck, 1997; Shaffer, 1997). Bone strength index[2] also was found to be lower in recruits with fracture compared with those without fracture. Another important predictor of fracture risk is the rate at which bone is being lost (Beck, 1997). The faster bone is lost, the more likely it is that undue mechanical stress can lead to fracture. The rate at which bone is lost is, in itself, an independent risk for fracture, as documented by studies of states of rapid bone loss such as those that occur after organ transplantation (Shane et al., 1997).

---

[1] Bone mineral density is bone mineral content, which is the amount of mineral at a particular skeletal site, divided by the area of the scanned region. BMD and bone mineral content are both measured by a variety of related technologies including dual energy x-ray absorptiometry.

[2] Bone strength index is based on the observation that the resistance of a bone to bending and twisting is directly related to the section modulus as measured by DXA and inversely related to bone length (Selker and Carter, 1989).

Kimmel and coworkers enrolled 3,300 female soldiers in a prospective study designed to determine predictors of stress fracture during basic combat training. Broadband ultrasound attenuation (BUA) of the bone (measurement using ultrasound techniques) was measured at baseline in all female soldiers and at the time of initial presentation with possible fracture. There were 338 soldiers with stress fractures. Fitness level at baseline, smoking history, and BUA were independent predictors of stress fracture risk, and those soldiers who developed fractures were found to have a greater decrease in BUA earlier in basic training than did soldiers who did not develop fractures. This decline in BUA during basic training indicates that soldiers respond to the additional bone stresses during this period with increased bone turnover, which causes transiently downward adjustment in bone strength due to an expansion of the remodeling space (Kimmel, 1997). Although BUA has been found to predict fracture risk in a group of individuals, current methodology cannot adequately assess individual risk for stress fracture due to its low sensitivity and specificity.

TECHNICAL MEASUREMENTS

As noted earlier, it is important to correlate results from bone imaging with clinical symptoms when diagnosing stress fractures. Other measures and techniques may be useful in the prediction of fracture risk, including the measurement of bone markers and bone mass.

Bone Markers

Bone markers are useful as indices of the dynamic processes of bone formation (osteocalcin, skeletal alkaline phosphatase, and type 1 procollagen carboxy-terminal extension peptide) and bone resorption (urinary hydroxyproline, total pyridinolines, and N-telopeptide) (Kleerekoper, 1997). They are helpful in gauging the extent of bone turnover, the net result of these two processes. Because high bone turnover in the adult is always associated with a net negative calcium balance, elevated bone markers usually signify bone loss. They can be useful as an adjunct to direct bone mass measurement, which is a static index. Recent studies suggest that bone markers may, in fact, be an independent predictor of bone loss and can be correlated with fracture risk. In addition, bone markers are used to monitor the course of therapy for osteoporosis. For instance, substantial reduction in markers of bone resorption with antiresorptive therapy for osteoporosis (e.g., estrogen, bisphosphonates, calcitonin) predicts subsequent increases in bone mass as determined by direct measurement.

The major limitations to the widespread use of these assays are the assays themselves, population variables, and day-to-day variability in the measurements. For changes to be helpful clinically, the results must exceed baseline values in general by greater than 30 percent. Nevertheless, bone markers are likely to become more useful as assay methods and collection procedures become more standardized.

Local events such as trauma, fragility, and stress fracture will increase bone remodeling at sites so challenged. The clinical presentation of stress fracture represents the cumulative effects of excess, repetitive mechanical forces applied to sites in the skeleton that are not competent to withstand such forces. The stress fracture is likely to be preceded by attempts at repair of the subclinical microdamage. Such repair mechanisms would involve activation of the remodeling processes normally associated with bone turnover. Using measurement of bone markers to detect these attempts at microrepair before fracture occurs has potential clinical value. However, it remains highly speculative whether such early events could be detected with the assays currently available, and it is unclear how such measurements would do more than call attention to such stresses on the skeleton. Such early indications of excessive mechanical stress would not necessarily eventuate in a clinical stress fracture.

Bone Mass

Of the wide variety of techniques available to measure bone mass, DXA is the most frequently used method, measuring total body as well as specific regions of bone. Since DXA involves measurement in only two dimensions, it does not provide a true estimate of density, the three-dimensional measurement (Beck et al., 1997). Quantitative computed tomography (QCT) is one method that measures true volumetric bone density, but it is limited in other ways (e.g., accuracy and radiation exposure). Methods employing ultrasound technology, still in the developmental phase, measure not only bone quantity, but also may incorporate a component of bone quality into the measurement (Kimmel et al., 1997). Thus, none of the current technologies—DXA, peripheral DXA (pDXA), QCT, peripheral QCT (pQCT) or ultrasound—can be used to screen for stress fractures. They are useful for bone density assessment, but there is scant literature to support the relationship between various levels of bone density and the risk of stress fractures.

Genetic Markers

An area of active investigation is a search for specific genes responsible for processes involved in the establishment of peak bone mass in youth and the progressive loss of bone mass with aging. Thus far, a number of candidate genes have been proposed. These include genes for the vitamin D receptor, the estrogen receptor, type 1 collagen, and IGF-1. The studies, which are still far from conclusive (Sambrook et al., 1996), nevertheless point clearly to a disorder that is likely to be polygenic, with a variety of genes contributing importantly to the osteoporotic process. Thus, each recruit brings to the field a different susceptibility to this condition and potentially a different susceptibility to fracture.

Diet

Adequate intakes of calcium and vitamin D are essential for optimizing bone health (IOM, 1997). Additionally, phosphorus, magnesium, and fluoride play a key role in the development and maintenance of bone. Other nutrients may have biological significance in the development and maintenance of bone, such as the microminerals copper, zinc, manganese, and boron and the vitamins C and K. However, calcium remains the most critical nutrient for bone development; the majority of the body's calcium resides in bone.

The recent Institute of Medicine Panel on Calcium and Related Nutrients used the maximal retention of calcium approach (the mathematical model that predicted the lowest level of calcium intake that maximized the amount of calcium retained in the body) for determining the adequate intake (AI) for calcium. This approach was used because increased calcium retention can be equated with higher bone mass as over 99 percent of total body calcium is found in bone (IOM, 1997, p. 4–13). The AI for calcium was an experimentally derived, approximate, group mean value for calcium that appears to support maximal calcium retention. An AI was considered for calcium, rather than an estimated average requirement (EAR[3]), due to: (1) uncertainties in the methods inherent in balance studies that were used to form the basis of the maximal retention model, (2) the lack of concordance between observational and experimental data, and (3) the lack of longitudinal data that could be used to verify the association of the experimentally derived calcium intakes for maximal retention with the rate and extent of long-term bone loss and its clinical sequelae, such as fracture (see IOM, 1997, p. S-4). The AI for calcium is 1,300 mg/d for 14 to 18 year olds and 1,000 mg/d for 19 to 30 year olds.

No consistent association has been found between the occurrence of stress fracture and calcium intake in either athletes or military recruits, possibly due to the relatively high calcium intakes in both groups (Bennell et al., 1996; Schwellnus and Jordaan, 1992). However, nutritional surveys of military women, as described in Table 2-1, reveal a wide range of calcium intakes that tend to be consistently lower in a number of different military facilities than the Military Recommended Dietary Allowances (MRDAs). One study in athletes found that calcium intakes greater than 800 mg/d were protective against stress fractures (Myburgh et al., 1990). Other investigators have found no association between stress fracture occurrence and calcium intakes of 1,100 mg/d (Bennell et al., 1996). Another study found no reduction in stress fractures in a group of military recruits given supplemental calcium, compared with those not receiving supplements, although the number in the supplemented group may have been too small to detect an effect (Schwellnus and Jordaan, 1992).

It is not known if dietary calcium requirements are increased during intense physical training. Decreased BMC was reported in trained male athletes in one report (Bilanin et al., 1989). Klesges et al. (1996), in a study of 11 National College Athletic Association Division I basketball players, reported a 6.1 percent decrease in total body BMC between the preseason and late summer, despite a mean intake of approximately 2,000 mg /d of calcium. The investigators attributed this loss of bone to negative calcium balance resulting from high calcium losses through sweat (mean of 247 mg/d). Although there was no control group in this study, a significant increase in BMC was observed the following year when the players were supplemented with varying doses of calcium (500–2,000 mg/d) and vitamin D (400–560 IU/d). The level of supplementation was matched to the degree of bone loss observed during the previous year. No

[3] The EAR is the nutrient intake value that is estimated to meet the requirement defined by a specified indicator of adequacy in 50 percent of the individuals in a life-stage and gender group.

TABLE 2-1 Military Nutritional Surveys: Mean Nutritional Intake of Female Soldiers

		Field		Dining Hall				
Nutrient	MRDA*	Hawaii 1985 *n* = 36	Bolivia 1990 *n* = 13	West Point 1979–1980 *n* = 54	Ft Jackson 1988 *n* = 40	West Point 1990 *n* = 86	Ft Jackson 1993 *n* = 49	Ft Sam Houston 1995 *n* = 50**
Energy, kcal	2,000–2,800	1,834	1,668	2,454	2,467	2,314	2,592	2,037
Protein, g	80	67	68	84	96	79	82	75
Carbohydrate, g	330	235	218	284	318	325	365	289
Fat, g	<93	70	57	107	94	81	94	63
Calcium, mg	800–1,200	577	664	954	907	1,001	728	918
Phosphorus, mg	800–1,200	1,065	1,059	1,347	1,600	1,391	1,296	1,333
Magnesium, mg	300	—	218	—	—	315	267	285
Iron, mg	18	11.9	11.7	16.2	18.4	28	16.2	16.8

* Military Recommend Dietary Allowance for moderately active military women aged 17–50 years.

** Officer basic training.

SOURCE: Adapted from King (1993).

other studies of calcium balance during intense physical activity could be identified. Loss of calcium through sweat has previously been reported to be low (40–144 mg/d) (Charles et al., 1991). The factorial approach[4] was used for estimating calcium requirements in adults aged 19 to 30 years (IOM, 1997) based on sweat losses obtained from a group of sedentary healthy volunteers (Charles et al., 1983), which averaged 63 mg/d over a 7-d period for both males and females. It is not known what the effects of prolonged, intense physical activity; stress; and altered eating patterns may have on calcium status in military women. Thus, further studies are needed to determine if physically active military women are at increased risk of not meeting their requirements for calcium due to increased loss of calcium in sweat.

Increased intakes of protein, sodium, and caffeine have been suggested to adversely affect calcium balance and optimal bone health (IOM, 1997, p. 4-4 to 4-5). However, there are no reports of an increased risk of stress fracture with increased intake of these food components or decreased intake of the other key bone-related nutrients (phosphorus, vitamin D, magnesium, and fluoride).

BODY COMPOSITION

Fat mass contributes to bone mineral mass, and thus to fracture risk, through at least two mechanisms. First, fat mass, through its influence on total body weight, has a trophic effect on bone mineral. Greater body fat and weight are linked with heavier skeletal mass, independent of gender or age (Chen et al., 1997), although fat mass or adipose tissue is not a main bone density determinant in young women. Second, fat mass or more specifically adipose tissue, is an important site of estrogen production in postmenopausal women (Rebuffe-Scrive et al., 1986). Estrogens positively influence bone mineral mass and density.

A well-established relationship also exists between skeletal muscle and bone mineral mass. In a classic study, Doyle et al. (1970) observed a significant correlation in human cadavers between vertebral bone mass and corresponding muscle. and Cohn (1975) extended these studies by demonstrating strong correlations at all ages between total body potassium, a measure of body cell mass, and total body calcium, a measure of bone mass. Burr (1997) examined the biomechanical link between skeletal muscle force or tension and corresponding bone mineral mass or density. According to Frost (as quoted by Burr), "voluntary muscle forces . . . dominate a bone's postnatal structural adaptations to mechanical usage." This link represents the classic biological relationship, "form follows function." These forces on bone are mainly transmitted by skeletal muscle tension and are not solely related to body weight. Forces generated by skeletal muscles appear to extend beyond generalized bone mineral effects; actual bone morphology and geometry are, to some extent, shaped by forces generated by skeletal muscles. Finally, as an example of the strong skeletal muscle–bone mineral association, quadriceps and hamstring skeletal muscle strength independently predict humerus and spine bone mineral density after controlling for such other relevant factors as

---

[4] "[A] more traditional factorial approach for estimating calcium requirements is to sum calcium needs for growth (accretion) plus calcium losses (urine, feces, and sweat) and adjust for absorption. Using this method, estimates for calcium requirements for adolescent girls and boys [aged 9–18 years] are 1,276 and 1,505 mg (31.9 and 37.6 mmol)/d, respectively" (IOM, 1997, p. 4–26). For females aged 19 to 30 years, the estimated requirement would be 1,393 mg (34.8 mmol)/d and for males, 1,437 mg (35.9 mmol)/d.

body weight (Brukner, 1997). Skeletal muscle strength-force relations are thought to influence bone mineral mass and density, although additional research on this topic is needed (Burr, 1997). Thus, fat mass and skeletal muscle mass, two body composition components extrinsic to the skeleton, appear to have important influences on the growth, mass, shape, geometry, and strength of bone.

Physical activities that generate a large muscle force can cause stress fractures at selected anatomic locations. For example, pelvic stress fractures involving the pubic rami that are often observed in women are thought to be related to excessive generated skeletal muscle force. Similarly, rowers and paddlers often suffer rib stress fractures (Matheson et al., 1987b). A related problem may occur in individuals who have a discrepancy in leg length. Discrepancies in contraction of skeletal muscles may cause an asymmetric load on bone that can produce a stress fracture (Matheson et al., 1987a). Several factors related to skeletal muscle mass and strength also favor inordinate bone loading and hence set the stage for stress fractures. Bones are encased in skeletal muscle, and muscles insulate bone and absorb mechanical loading. Muscle resists mechanical stress on bone, particularly some muscles that resist bending and torsion. For example, the tensor faciae latae muscle in the leg tends to resist bending of the femur and may transmit stresses resulting from bending (i.e., where bone is weaker to axial compression) at sites where the bone is stronger. Moreover, those individuals who have weaker muscles may fatigue more easily. The person's musculoskeletal system thereby has a reduced ability to resist continued bending and loading stresses. Inadequate skeletal muscle mass or strength may therefore favor transmission of unduly large forces to bone and thus permit development of stress fractures. In favor of this hypothesis, Brukner (1997) and Beck et al. (1996) observed reduced calf girth in women who suffered stress fractures during basic combat training. Although the conclusion is not clearly documented, smaller male soldiers are at greater risk of stress fracture than are larger male soldiers, and this increased risk may stem from either their reduced skeletal muscle mass or poorer physical conditioning.

PHYSICAL ACTIVITY AND FITNESS

Numerous cross-sectional studies in athletes have supported an association between BMD and long-term exercise behaviors (see review article, Suominen, 1993). In general, the increases in BMD appear to be specific to the regions that are being loaded (Alfredson et al., 1996; Taafe et al., 1997), and the effect appears to be long term (Etherington et al., 1996).

Although the concept that weight-bearing activity determines the shape and mass of bone is generally accepted, results from controlled trials of physical activity in nonathletes are not consistent. A recent review of prospective trials of predominantly older women showed that a beneficial effect of increased activity on BMD was observed in those groups of individuals consuming a mean calcium intake greater than 1,100 mg/d of calcium. Results of trials in groups of individuals consuming less than 1,100 mg/d tended to show no benefit of activity on BMD (Specker, 1996). No prospective controlled study specifically designed to test the hypothesis that calcium intake modifies the bone response to activity has been reported.

The term *fitness* has several meanings. In the first context, fitness refers to the level of cardiorespiratory reserve (aerobic capacity), and in the second, it refers to a more general readiness to participate in physical activity. The latter context includes adaptations such as muscular strength, skill development, and musculoskeletal readiness. From the previous section on pathophysiology of stress fractures, it is clear that to avoid cumulative microdamage to bone, the rate of loading must closely match the rate of remodeling. However, unlike a low level of aerobic fitness in which the person is simply unable to complete a physical task at a higher intensity until metabolic and cardiorespiratory adaptations are sufficient, even sedentary people can tolerate a large volume of cyclic loading to their skeletal system for a period of several weeks before symptoms of stress fracture occur. The architectural adaptations to bone that permit cyclic loading at higher levels of physical activity are not required in the first few weeks of training, and any excessive strain produced during this early phase does not impair a person's ability to participate until such time as the cumulative stress produces clinically obvious symptoms. Thus, to attain fitness, a training program must include a history of sufficient loading and remodeling within bone if stress injuries and fractures are to be prevented during periods of intense training.

The mechanical and cellular response of bone to loading is based on four factors: (1) the number of strain cycles experienced by the bone (volume of training, total cumulative load), (2) the frequency of strain cycles or load per unit time (the intensity, pace, time for recovery), (3) magnitude of strain of each load cycle (factors that affect shock absorption and shock attenuation include muscular strength and endurance, footwear, and lower extremity alignment factors), and (4) duration of each strain cycle (terrain, lower extremity alignment).

From a clinical perspective, there are five factors that contribute to stress fracture occurrence.

1. Training errors are increases in physical activity (loading) at a rate that exceeds the bone's rate of remodeling. The expression "too much too soon" includes all components of training such as volume, intensity, pace, and recovery. This is the single factor most likely to cause a stress fracture in a nonelite, recreational athlete or a recruit in basic military training (Matheson et al., 1987a).

2. Muscle fatigue is also an important factor. Attenuation of ground reaction forces principally through eccentric contraction of muscle minimizes the load transmitted directly to bone. If muscle fatigue occurs during an exercise bout, bone will experience a greater load. Clinical measurement of muscular strength does not measure muscle fatigue, which is the metabolic capability to produce adenosine triphosphate (ATP) continuously through oxidative phosphorylation at the rate required to sustain a given workload. Resistance to fatigue only occurs through sport-specific training, and muscular adaptations that provide enhanced oxidative capacity take from 8 to 16 weeks to develop fully (Matheson et al., 1987a).

3. Lower extremity alignment predisposes a person to the development of stress fractures. High arched, *pes cavus*-style feet absorb less shock, while *pes planus* ("flat foot") feet transmit more force to the tibia. *Genu varum* (angled inward or knock-kneed) and *valgum* (angled outward or bowlegged), excessive Q angles (the angle of intersection between the direction of pull on the patella by the quadriceps muscles and the direction of resistance by the patellar tendon), leg length discrepancies, and femoral neck anteversion are all associated with variations in gait that can influence the distribution of forces to bone in the lower extremity (Matheson et al., 1987a).

4. Terrain influences force delivered to bone in two ways. Hard surfaces require greater shock absorption by lower leg muscles, and cambered or uneven surfaces require compensatory muscular contractions that alter the balance of loading between the two lower extremities.

5. Equipment, particularly footwear, can influence the load delivered to bone both with respect to shock absorption and whether the design accommodates the foot type and lower extremity alignment. Guidelines for selecting appropriate footwear are provided in the Army's *Physical Fitness Training* manual (FM 21-20, 1992), and recruits are often provided assistance in making the correct selection based on a screening exam they receive in their unit.

A well-designed shoe (flexible soles, shock absorbing, good arch and heel support) can assist in reducing the number of lower limb injuries arising from sport and training activities. However, it has been reported that a training shoe is rarely implicated in a stress fracture injury (Nike, 1987). In the military, the general trend has been to employ athletic shoes rather than boots for physical training sessions, particularly for running, at least during the early stages of recruit training. Current U.S. Army training policy (Bentley, 1978) allows running shoes rather than military combat boots to be worn during training runs. This policy has been supported by a study in New Zealand Army recruits (Stacy and Hungeford, 1984). These investigators found that total injuries were reduced from 85 per 100 to 52 per 100 recruits by eliminating running in boots during the first 5 weeks and by gradually introducing boots progressively over this period. Comparisons between training shoes and combat boots have shown that boots are almost 50 percent worse in rear foot shock absorption, 100 percent less flexible, and 200 percent less shock absorbent in the forefoot (Cavanagh, 1980). Approximately one-third of the recruit's training time is spent in a running shoe (personal communication, L. Tomasi, Ft. Benning, 1998).

Because injuries can be caused by running on hard surfaces, soldiers should, if possible, avoid running on concrete. Asphalt surfaces provide more cushioning than concrete. Soft, even surfaces are best for injury prevention such as grass paths, dirt paths, or park trails. However, with adequate footwear and recovery periods, running on roads and other hard surfaces should pose no problem. Fine-tuning of athletic footwear to specific foot types can also be helpful. The high arch, rigid, *pes cavus* foot benefits from a flexible shoe with a curved last and excellent shock-absorbing characteristics. The flexible *pes planus* style of foot benefits from a straight-sole shoe with a stiff heel counter that provides motion control.

ORAL CONTRACEPTIVES

Several investigators have shown an increase in BMD with oral contraceptive use in premenopausal women (Fortney et al., 1994; Goldsmith and Johnston, 1975; Lindsay et al., 1986; Recker et al., 1992; Shargil 1985) and past use in postmenopausal women (Enzelsberger et al., 1988; Goldsmith and Johnston, 1975; Kleerekoper et al., 1991; Kritz-Silverstein and Barrett-Connor, 1993), while others have failed to detect a beneficial effect on bone in premenopausal (Hall et al., 1990; Hreshchyshyn et al., 1988; Mazes and Barden, 1991; Murphy et al., 1993; Volpe et al., 1993) and postmenopausal women (Hreshchyshyn et al., 1988; Murphy et al., 1993). This discrepancy in results can be explained, at least in part by different dosages and durations of pill use, varying ages of the population, varying lengths of follow-up, insufficient sample size, inadequate control for confounders, and different bone sites and techniques for measurement of BMD (DeCherney, 1996; Garnero et al., 1995).

Consistent evidence supports a causal relationship between estrogen deficiency and osteoporosis and the efficacy of estrogen replacement therapy in reducing bone loss after cessation of ovarian function following oophorectomy, premature ovarian failure, and menopause (Mehta, 1993). However, important differences in the formulation of drugs, dosage, and regimen exist among studies evaluating hormone replacement therapy and oral contraceptives use.

In retrospective epidemiological studies, women who used oral contraceptives for greater than 10 years had the greatest protection against low BMD (Enzelsberger et al., 1988; Kleerekoper et al., 1991). In a cross-sectional study of premenopausal women taking 30 μg ethinyl estradiol for a mean duration of 6.7 years, all markers of bone formation (serum osteocalcin, bone-specific alkaline phosphatase, C-terminal propeptide of type 1 collagen) and resorption (pyridinoline cross-linked peptides) were decreased (Garnero et al., 1995). However, total body BMC and BMD, and lumbar spine, total hip, and distal radius BMD did not differ between oral contraceptive users and nonusers.

During the 20 years that combined estrogen-progestagen preparations have been used, the dosage has been modified to reduce side effects and complications. Most compounds now include 35 μg or less of estrogen and varying amounts of progestagen. The advent of very low dose oral contraceptives (< 20 μg/d) has reduced the thrombotic complications.

Progestogenic components of oral contraceptives may have a positive impact on BMD, although evidence is less conclusive. Progestational agents such as Norethindrone have estrogen-like properties and interact with androgen receptors. Urinary calcium excretion was reduced and bone mass was stabilized or increased with use of certain progestational agents alone or in combination with estrogen (Riis et al., 1990; Stevenson et al., 1990; Surrey et al., 1990).

Exogenous estrogen-progestagen hormones given to women of reproductive status may positively affect peak bone mass reached in adulthood and the rate of premenopausal bone loss, both of which are important for future fracture risks. In contrast, long-acting progestagens used alone may have a detrimental effect on BMD. Depot medroxyprogesterone acetate (Depo-Provera), an injectable long-acting progestagen, inhibits gonadotropin secretion and results in a relative estrogen-deficiency state. Disruption of menstrual cycling is common, with an incidence of 55 percent amenorrhea after 12 months of treatment and 68 percent after 24 months. In a cross-sectional study, 30 women using Depo-Provera for more than 5 years had decreased BMD at the lumbar spine and femoral neck compared with premenopausal women not using the preparation (Cundy et al., 1991).

A 6-mo prospective, randomized trial comparing Depo-Provera with subdermal implanted progestin levonorgestral treatment (Norplant) was conducted in 22 premenopausal women, ages 20 to 45 years (Naessen et al., 1995). Forearm BMD increased 2.9 percent with Norplant and was stable with Depo-Provera treatment. Depo-Provera increased bone turnover, and Norplant increased bone formation as evidenced by increased serum alkaline phosphatase, osteocalcin, and estradiol. The duration of the trial may not have been long enough to observe the adverse effects of Depo-Provera that have been seen in other studies.

Thus, the data suggest there are no detrimental effects of oral estrogen-containing contraceptives on bone health, and in fact, they may afford protection from loss of bone in some women. Because of the small, but significant increased risk of breast cancer with unopposed estrogen therapy, estrogen-progesterone replacement therapy combinations should be used. The use of various estrogen analogs such as Droloxifene or Raloxifine, which antagonize the oncogenic effect of estrogen, offer promise for future research. Not enough is known yet about whether progestational agents, when used alone for contraception, will lead to bone loss.

OTHER LIFESTYLE FACTORS

Both smoking and alcohol are moderately associated with increased risk of fracture (Slemenda et al., 1989). Smoking is associated with lower body weight, earlier menopause, and lower postmenopausal estrogen levels, factors that each carry a risk of stress fractures (Heaney, 1996). The results of a recent meta-analysis noted an increased risk of hip fracture with cigarette smoking in postmenopausal women, which increased with increasing age (Law and Hackshaw, 1997). However, fracture risk did not increase with smoking in premenopausal women, and smokers were found to have similar BMD to nonsmokers.

In a study of women during Army BCT, Westphal et al. (1995) noted that the consumption of alcohol appeared to be an independent risk factor for injuries, as a significant dose response was found for time-loss injuries in women who successively reported more days of alcohol consumption compared with nondrinkers. It is not known what percentage of these injuries were due to stress fractures and whether they might have been related to alcohol consumption. Alcohol abuse impairs the absorption, utilization, storage, and excretion of nutrients, which, in combination with inadequate intake, results in nutritionally compromised conditions. Excess alcohol consumption is often associated with low dairy food intake and, additionally, is a cause of hypercalciuria (Heaney, 1996). It is likely that high blood alcohol levels are directly toxic to osteoblasts (Laitinen and Valimaki, 1991). Increased alcohol use has been shown to be marginally associated with increased risk of fracture (Slemenda et al., 1992).

In a study performed by McDermott (1996), a survey was conducted in 1,000 premenopausal military women to assess dietary calcium intakes, physical activity, and habits affecting skeletal health. In a subset of 90 women who completed bone density testing by DXA, the attainment of peak bone mass was unaffected by history of smoking, alcohol, and caffeine use during high school.

SUMMARY

Stress fracture represents the cumulative effects of repetitive mechanical loading at a rate greater than that of osteoblastic new bone formation. Disruption of this remodeling balance leads to symptomatic microfracture, which if untreated, may progress to complete fracture.

Measurements of bone mass or density are predictive of fracture risk in postmenopausal women, but data on the relationship between BMD and stress fracture are less plentiful. Current methods for the assessment of bone mass presently are not suitable to screen for stress fractures. Preliminary data suggest that the mean BMD of military recruits who suffer a stress fracture is lower than that of recruits not suffering a stress fracture (Beck, 1997). In addition, elite athletes with stress fractures have lower BMD than athletes without stress fractures (Bennell et al., 1996). However, both the fracture and nonfracture groups of military recruits and athletes had BMD measurements within the normal range. Moreover, except for rare instances where stress fractures result from an underlying metabolic bone disorder, there currently is no evidence that the risk of developing osteoporosis is increased in individuals who previously suffered a stress fracture.

Fat mass and skeletal muscle mass have important influences on bone that affect its growth, total mass, shape, geometry and strength. While skeletal muscles insulate bone and absorb mechanical loading, excessive muscular development can generate large muscle force and may cause stress fractures at selected anatomic locations.

Regular participation in physical activity develops muscular strength, skill and readiness. The rate of loading must closely match the rate of bone remodeling in order to prevent injuries and stress fractures during BCT. Muscle fatigue, lower extremity alignment, terrain, and equipment are other key factors that contribute to the occurrence of stress fractures (Matheson et al., 1987a).

Other factors that may influence the risk of stress fractures are exogenous estrogen-progestagen hormones given to women of reproductive age. These synthetic hormones may positively affect peak bone mass reached in adulthood and the rate of postmenopausal bone loss, both of which are important risks for future fracture. In contrast, long-acting progestagens may have a detrimental effect on BMD (Naessen et al., 1995).

3

Effects of Caloric Intake, Physical Activity and Hormonal Factors on Bone Health

CALORIC/HORMONAL FACTORS

Women in the military may be placed in situations or under conditions that are not optimal for the accrual or maintenance of peak bone mass. Conditions that induce estrogen deficiency from any cause, whether hormonal or due to caloric insufficiency, may adversely affect the skeleton. In military women, there is cause for concern about hypothalamic amenorrhea due to physical or emotional stress, excessive exercise and/or eating disorders, therapy with gonadotropin-releasing hormone (GnRH) agonists for the treatment of endometriosis, and the use of contraceptives that prevent menstruation; all of these factors may lower BMD and increase the risk for stress fractures. A decrease in hypothalamic GnRH leads to anovulation and increased bone resorption due to decreased estradiol secretion. Because military women are now eligible for most military occupational specialties, an increase in the time they spend in arduous, physically demanding situations may increase the incidence of hypothalamic amenorrhea. Women may eventually be eligible for participation in the Ranger training program[1], in which soldiers are subjected to severe energy restriction.

Concern about adhering to existing military standards for body weight and composition also may lead to disordered eating patterns[2] that are known to adversely affect women's long-term bone health. Although exact numbers are not available for the military population, dietary energy restriction to maintain "optimal" body weight is common in the civilian population, and young women entering the military may already be involved in chronic dietary practices that may negatively influence their nutrient and hormonal status and thereby their bone health (IOM, 1998).

Effects of Low Energy Intake on Hormonal Levels and Bone Health

The impact of low energy intake on the hormonal milieu in young women of military age is well documented. Kurzer and Calloway (1985) showed that a decrease in energy intake to 43 percent of need for only 1 month resulted in menstrual abnormalities in two of six subjects, with decreases in circulating estrogen and progesterone. Hypoestrogenemia or luteal suppression (shortened luteal phase of the menstrual cycle with reduction in progesterone secretion) was also found in female athletes (ACSM, 1997), in whom high energy outputs are often coupled with lower than expected energy intakes (Mulligan and Butterfield, 1990). Female athletes who are amenorrheic also demonstrated suppressed insulin release (Laughlin et al., 1994), elevated growth hormone (Laughlin et al., 1994), mildly elevated cortisol levels (Loucks, 1989) in conjunction with low tri-iodothyronine (T3) (Loucks et al., 1992), and high levels of IGF-1 binding protein (Laughlin et al., 1994), all of which may adversely affect bone turnover and the accrual of peak bone mass. Several investigators have documented low bone mass in young women athletes, especially those who are amenorrheic (Drinkwater et al., 1984) and have low energy intakes (Marcus et al., 1985).

The complete etiology of the hormonal changes that may accompany strenuous athletic activity is unknown. (The decrease in luteal phase length has been associated with a reduction in luteinizing hormone [LH] pulsatility and an increase in pulse height, a response thought to originate at the level of the hypothalamus [Loucks, 1996] via changes in the pulsatile secretions of GnRH.) However, the interactions resulting in decreased GnRH pulsatility are unknown.

Loucks and colleagues (1989) have shown that the disrupted LH pulsatility is present in normally menstruating female athletes as well as those who are amenorrheic and have proposed the concept of decreased energy availability to explain this and other aspects of the syndrome. They speculate that the disruption in menstrual function that accompanies exercise is akin to that

---

[1] The U.S. Army Ranger training program is a physically and psychologically demanding program used by the Army to screen male officers and enlisted soldiers for entry into special operations units. The training consists of three 3-wk phases conducted at widely varying sites with differing physical demands: military base training, mountain training, and swamp training.

[2] Disordered eating describes a wide spectrum of harmful behaviors in a continuum between over- and undereating where abnormal measures are taken to control weight (e.g., bingeing, purging, dieting, and restricting food intake) (ACSM, 1997).

associated with fasting or starvation, where energy intake is insufficient to meet metabolic demands (Loucks, 1996).

The concept of energy availability is based on the understanding that mammals divide their energy intake among a variety of energy-requiring functions, including cellular maintenance, thermoregulation, motor activity, growth, reproduction, and storage, with this order representing the hierarchy of function (Wade and Schneider, 1992). When energy intake is limited, functions at the top of the hierarchy are performed at the expense of those at the bottom. Thus, optimal menstrual function requires a minimal amount of available energy. When activity is high, the energy available for menstrual function may be compromised unless energy intake is appropriately adjusted.

At the workshop, Loucks (1997) presented data illustrating her attempts to dissect the relationship between activity level and energy intake in order to explain this phenomenon. In a series of short-term and acute studies (4–5 days in duration) in eumenorrheic sedentary women (Loucks and Callister, 1993) and eumenorrheic active women (Loucks et al., 1994), in whom exercise and energy intake were manipulated to limit energy availability, even this short period of low energy availability resulted in changes in LH pulsatility and suppression of T3 levels. She has also demonstrated that exercise has no further effect beyond that of decreasing energy availability (Loucks and Callister, 1993). The suppression of T3 and the changes in LH pulsatility occurred at a threshold level of energy availability (operationally defined as dietary energy intake minus exercise energy expenditure) of 20 to 25 kcal/kg lean body mass in women (Loucks and Heath, 1994). Unpublished data presented at the workshop suggested that a similar low energy availability in men resulted in no change in LH pulsatility, although other endocrine changes were similar to those seen in women.

In additional experiments on physically active women, Williams et al. (1995) have shown similar results. Active eumenorrheic women experienced suppressed LH pulsatility after only 3 days of training when dietary energy intake was reduced. This condition reversed itself when the dietary intake was appropriately increased.

Further support for the concept that the hormonal changes accompanying amenorrhea in female athletes derive from low energy availability comes from the report of Dueck et al. (1996). In a pilot study, they evaluated LH pulsatility and cortisol secretion in three eumenorrheic women athletes as compared with the same parameters in an amenorrheic athlete. This athlete was treated by increasing energy intake by approximately 350 kcal/d and decreasing training by 1 d/wk, with an increase in net energy availability of about 250 kcal/d. At the end of 15 weeks, all athletes were again tested. In the previously amenorrheic athlete, LH pulsatility had returned to match the normal pattern, cortisol secretion had fallen to within normal limits, and normal menstrual function had returned.

Effect of Dieting and Weight Loss on Bone Health

Independent of menstrual dysfunction, weight loss may decrease BMD. Substantial weight loss due to reduced energy intake in overweight postmenopausal women was associated with a significant loss of total-body BMD (Compston et al., 1992; Jensen et al., 1994; Svendsen et al., 1993). In young women, moderate dieting at a level of 27 percent energy restriction resulted in a

3.4 kg weight loss, a 0.7 percent decrease in total-body BMD, and a 0.5 percent decrease in lumbar spine BMD (Ramsdale and Bassey, 1994). However, the above studies examining the effect of weight loss on bone mineral should be interpreted cautiously, because changes in total-body bone mineral measured by older software versions of DXA instruments may have been erroneous if considerable change in soft tissue composition occurred (Svendsen et al., 1993).

Incidence of Caloric Restriction and Disordered Eating Patterns in Military Women

Because stress fractures occur primarily during basic training, it would be useful to know the dietary practices of women who enter into the military to determine if caloric restriction and disordered eating patterns are related to the incidence of stress fractures. Most reports of diagnosed eating disorders in the civilian population place the incidence of anorexia nervosa at 0.5 to 1 percent by the *Diagnostic and Statistical Manual of Mental Disorders,* 4th edition (DSM-IV, 1994) criteria and that of bulimia nervosa at 1 to 4 percent of the women studied. Others have suggested that subclinical eating disorders are significantly more prevalent in the 18- to 24-year old age group (Beals and Manore, 1994; Sundgot-Borgan, 1993). Clinical eating disorders appear to be rare among military women, but representative data are not available on the prevalence of disordered eating patterns among these women. Interpretation of data from the military is complicated by the policy that, until recently, defined eating disorders as grounds for dismissal (IOM, 1998). Thus, attempts to assess disordered eating of any kind in the past have been inadequate and probably have underestimated the problem. However, the emphasis on appearance, which is formalized in DoD documents (U.S. Department of Defense Directive 1308.1, 1995; U.S. Department of Defense Directive 1308.3, 1995, U.S. Department of the Army AR 600-9, 1986), is a risk factor for development of such conditions. The *Perception of Wellness and Readiness Assessment* (POWR'95) of Navy and Marine Corps personnel, conducted in 1995, employed questions from the *Eating Disorders Inventory,* a validated tool that has been shown to have predictive value in assessing risk of disordered eating (Garner and Olmstead, 1991). POWR'95 revealed that 11 percent of women respondents used diet pills to lose or maintain weight, 13 percent ate in secret, and 50 percent were dissatisfied with their weight. These three factors are most predictive of disordered eating (especially bulimia) (Hourani, 1996). Respondents to this same survey indicated a 1.5 percent incidence of bulimia at some time in their lives and a 1.2 percent incidence at the time of the survey. In a recent report by Lauder (1997), 33.6 percent of 423 active-duty women in the Army were judged to be at risk for disordered eating, and 8 percent fulfilled the criteria for disordered eating. Fewer than 1 percent had anorexia nervosa or bulimia. As mentioned above, these data may significantly underestimate the incidence of these eating patterns in the military. A similar study of Navy midshipmen answering similar questions suggested that 10 percent of the women and 3.5 percent of the men were at risk for disordered eating patterns (Drake, 1996).

Results of these surveys as well as others (*Survey of Health Related Behaviors among Military Personnel*, 1995; *Survey of Nutrition Knowledge of Active-Duty Navy Personnel*, 1990) have suggested that the prevalence of overweight among active-duty women is at least comparable to that of a similar population of civilian women. Service-wide, 25 to 50 percent of the women surveyed reported that they exceeded the weight standards set for their own branch of the service. However, the surveys also demonstrated that the percentage of active-duty women who are dieting and/or dissatisfied with their weight[3] (40–80% in the regular forces) is significantly higher than the percentage of women who are actually overweight. In young recruits participating in basic training or in the U.S. Military Academy at West Point, the percentage of women dieting was equally high (60% and 74%, respectively), which suggests an early establishment of a food intake pattern that might jeopardize bone health (Klicka et al., 1993). The requirement to meet military weight standards every 6 months may induce "crash" or chronic dieting and weight cycling (repetitive episodes of weight loss followed by weight gain). In addition, the activity level that accompanies, first, basic training and, then, the day-to-day activities of a fighting soldier (Army women have been estimated to expend 1,300 kcal/d in exercise [Hourani, 1996]) may put the female soldier at continued risk of amenorrhea. Drake (1996) reported that 10 to 15 percent of female midshipmen become oligomenorrheic within the first year at the U.S. Naval Academy, and 5 to 6 percent develop full amenorrhea. Lauder (1997) reported that among 423 active-duty women, 2.2 and 3.3 percent were amenorrheic and oligomenorrheic, respectively, excluding women on hormonal birth control.

Hypothalamic Amenorrhea and Bone Health

Premature bone demineralization occurs in women with hypothalamic amenorrhea and oligomenorrhea associated with eating disorders and strenuous physical activity. This complex syndrome has been referred to as the *female athlete triad* (ACSM, 1997; Bennell et al., 1995). In young women with amenorrhea associated with weight loss, BMD loss occurs soon after amenorrhea develops. Hypoestrogenic amenorrhea has been correlated with the age of onset of menstruation, the duration of amenorrhea, and low body fat mass. Although fat stores are an important component of energy balance, there is no convincing evidence that body fat has a direct causal role in regulating ovulation (Loucks, 1996).

In a randomized trial, 24 young women with hypothalamic amenorrhea or oligomenorrhea were treated with oral contraceptives, medroxyprogesterone, or a placebo for 12 months (Hergenroeder et al., 1997). In amenorrheic subjects receiving oral contraceptives, lumbar spine, and total BMC and BMD were higher at 12 months compared with those on medroxyprogesterone, or the placebo. In oligomenorrheic subjects treated with medroxyprogesterone, no detectable improvement in BMD was seen.

In another randomized trial, 48 amenorrheic young women with anorexia nervosa received estrogen and progestin, or no replacement, and were re-evaluated 18 months later (Klibanski et al., 1995). No significant change was seen in BMD in the treated versus the placebo group; however, a 4 percent increase in BMD was observed in treated patients whose initial body weight was less than 70 percent of ideal. Despite this partial protection, estrogen and progestin administration did not reverse the osteopenia seen in these young, amenorrheic women, which emphasizes the multifactorial etiology of the anorexia syndrome. Energy restriction, low body weight, body fat

---

3 Based on self-reported weights and heights (IOM, 1998), the prevalence rates for underweight (BMI < 19.0) ranged from 3.6 percent for Navy women to 6.8 percent for Marine Corps women.

depletion, and nutritionally dependent hormones (i.e., hormones such as thyroid, cortisol, GH, and IGF-1 whose synthesis or secretion is dependent on energy-protein intake) together with the steroid hormones interact to influence BMD.

Possible Effects of Excessive Exercise on Bone Health

In general, exercise promotes bone mineralization, but the beneficial effect of exercise on BMD can be lost, and significant bone loss can result if exercise training is excessive (Hergenroeder, 1995). Regular recreational exercise at or above a basic conditioning level does not increase infertility or disturb the menstrual cycle, but abrupt, large changes in exercise frequency or intensity, or excessive exercise resulting in weight loss, can disturb menstrual function, resulting in hypoestrogenic amenorrhea, anovulatory cycles, and luteal phase deficiency (Clapp and Little, 1995). A strenuous running program in untrained women with normal cycles induced menstrual disturbance within 1 month in the majority of subjects (Bullen et al., 1985). Although not a prerequisite for bone loss, the additional stress of body weight loss, superimposed during the training program, increased the severity and frequency of menstrual changes. Estrogen production, not progesterone, appears to be the most important hormone in maintaining bone mass in women with menstrual cycle disturbances, such as short luteal cycle (De Souza, 1997). Subtle disturbances associated with running such as decreased follicular phase estradiol also appear to be related to bone loss.

Reductions in circulating estrogens characteristic of the female athlete triad are of clinical concern. The extent to which amenorrhea limits the skeletal response to mechanical loading is not clear. In postmenopausal women, resistance training combined with hormone replacement therapy led to substantial and unprecedented rises in vertebral BMD (Notelovitz et al., 1991). In another study of amenorrheic runners, those receiving hormone replacement therapy increased bone density during training, while those not receiving treatment did not experience an increase in bone density (Cumming, 1996).

Vigorous exercise, hypogonadism, and leanness in women with athletic amenorrhea may not be associated with generalized osteoporosis. Young and colleagues (1994) studied 44 ballet dancers with amenorrhea or oligomenorrhea, 18 sedentary amenorrheic girls with anorexia nervosa, and 23 girls with regular menstrual cycles. BMD was normal or elevated at weight-bearing sites (trochanter) in dancers, and it was normal or reduced at these sites in sedentary amenorrheic girls. BMD at non-weightbearing sites was reduced in dancers, similar to sedentary amenorrheic girls. Weight-bearing exercise may offset effects of hypogonadism at predominantly cortical weight-bearing sites such as proximal femur. Nonweight-bearing sites with substantial trabecular bone, such as lumbar spine, may be adversely affected by hypogonadism. Resumption of menses in athletes results in a gain in bone density; however, their values are still less than that of eumenorrheic counterparts. As the length of the amenorrheic period is prolonged, bone loss can occur at weight-bearing sites that are largely cortical bone (Rencken, 1996).

SUMMARY

Conditions that induce estrogen deficiency from any cause, such as energy insufficiency either as a result of dieting or excessive physical activity, may adversely affect bone health. Whether continued disruption leads to the phenomenon of athletic amenorrhea is not known; however, normal reproductive hormone secretion can be reinstated in amenorrheic women athletes simply by increasing the energy intake. Some of the hormonal changes of athletic amenorrhea are similar to those created by imposing a state of low energy availability on sedentary or active women, namely, suppression of T3 secretion and alteration in LH pulsatility. In addition, it has been shown that abnormal cortisol secretion associated with the amenorrhea (which may negatively influence bone health) can also be corrected by increasing energy intakes. Oral contraceptives may also afford protection from loss of bone minerals in some women

The extent to which amenorrhea limits the skeletal response to mechanical loading is not clear. In general, exercise promotes bone mineralization, but the beneficial effect of exercise on BMD can be lost, and significant bone loss can result if exercise training is not matched by adequate caloric intake.

The prevalence of overweight among active-duty women is at least comparable to that of a similar population of civilian women. A large percentage of military women surveyed reported that they exceeded weight standards, and even a larger percentage reported they are dieting or dissatisfied with their weight (IOM, 1998).

Premature bone demineralization occurs in women with hypothalamic amenorrhea and oligomenorrhea associated with eating disorders as well as with strenuous physical activity. Eating disorders are rare among military women; however, representative data are not available on the prevalence of disordered eating patterns among military women. In a recent report, one-third of the Army active-duty women studied were documented to be at risk of disordered eating, and 8 percent fulfilled the criteria for disordered eating.

4

Conclusions and Recommendations

RESPONSE TO TASK QUESTIONS

1. Why is the incidence of stress fractures in military combat training greater for women than for men?

Stress fracture rates among female military trainees during basic training are more than twice those reported for males. This greater incidence appears to be due in part to the initial entry level of fitness of the recruits and specifically the ability of bone to withstand the sudden large increase in physical loading. Some studies that controlled for aerobic fitness were unable to demonstrate a difference in the incidence of injury between males and females when individuals of the same fitness level were compared. Factors such as increased stride length (shorter women having the same stride length as tall men in "co-ed" marching situations) and variations in specific exercise activities (different loading force during drop-knee push-ups) may contribute to the different site distribution of stress fractures in military women compared with men. When training regimens are imposed to deliver the necessary level of physical fitness to meet standards, the resultant stress on the less physically fit (usually women) increases the likelihood of injury. According to military fitness experts, the fitness level of all new recruits has been decreasing over the past years. Reversing the trend in fitness in recruits may require setting higher and more relevant standards for entry. Preventing injury once recruits are in basic training may require reassessing methods used to achieve the desired improvement in fitness. A careful analysis of methods designed to achieve the desired degree of physical fitness during basic training without incurring an excessive injury rate with its associated loss of training time seems appropriate at this time.

2. What is the relationship of genetics and body composition to bone density and the incidence of stress fractures in women?

Genetics is a determinant of peak bone mass, but it is not known what genes are important, nor is it known how prominent they are in the risk assessment profile for stress fractures. Body mass and composition per se influence bone density. Greater body mass is associated with higher levels of bone mineral mass and density. Hence, individuals who are heavier and have a larger and denser skeleton are at lower risk of bone fracture, particularly osteoporosis-related fractures.

Stress fractures are associated not only with reduced skeletal muscle mass and its concomitant increased fatigability and lower fitness levels but also with an excessive skeletal muscle mass and its enhanced strength. Reduced skeletal muscle mass with associated lower strength and greater fatigability may limit the ability of muscle to decrease bone stress. This relationship between small muscle mass and increased bone fragility may account for the observed association between lower calf circumference and stress fracture risk in women. Bone stress created by excessive or rapid incremental skeletal muscle contraction and loading forces can cause fractures at specific anatomic sites.

In sum, body mass and composition play a substantial role in establishing an individual's skeletal properties including ability to stimulate bone growth and turnover and to withstand physical demands that predispose to stress fracture.

3. What are the effects of diet, physical activity, contraceptive use, and other lifestyle factors (smoking and alcohol) on the accrual of peak bone mineral content, incidence of stress fractures, and development of osteoporosis in military women?

Energy intake by military women should be adequate (2,000–2,800 kcal/d) to maintain weight during moderate and intensive physical fitness training. A diet adequate in calcium, phosphorus, magnesium, and vitamin D (as defined by IOM, 1997) and moderate in sodium and protein (NRC, 1989) should optimize bone health in the short term and theoretically should reduce the long-term risk of developing osteoporosis.

A healthy, active lifestyle should reduce further the long-term risk for osteoporosis. Physical activity of a weight-bearing nature should be introduced in a gradual and progressive manner to minimize risk of stress fractures. The use of oral contraceptives that contain estrogen with or without progestational agents are not considered to have long-term detrimental effects on women's bone health. Some studies show, in fact, that the use of such agents might have a positive impact on the developing young female skeleton. In contrast, the use of long-acting, depot preparations of progestational agents, like medroxyprogestrerone (Depo-Provera) has been associated with relative estrogen deficiency and reduced bone mass.

Gonadotropin-releasing hormone (GnRH) agonists used to treat endometriosis (Lupron) interfere with the hypothalamic-pituitary-ovarian axis, inducing a state of estrogen deficiency. Long-term use of such GnRH agonists is of concern because (1) it mimics the menopausal state of estrogen deficiency, and (2) it has been associated with bone loss.

Agents used to treat the pain and inflammation of injury can include steroids and nonsteroidal anti-inflammatory agents (NSAIDs). Because of the potential of steroids to induce bone loss by the many mechanisms described earlier in this report, their use should be restricted to special circumstances, short time periods, and the lowest possible doses. An attractive alternative are the NSAIDs, which should not harbor the same potential for negative effects on bone as do the steroidal agents.

Cigarette smoking may be a risk factor for the long-term risk of osteoporosis, whereas excessive alcohol consumption may be a risk factor in the short term for overall injuries. Whether these lifestyle factors are directly related to the development of stress fractures in the short term or are indirectly related through their long-term influence on bone density is not known.

4. How do caloric restriction and disordered eating patterns affect hormonal balance and the accrual and maintenance of peak bone mineral content?

Energy restriction adversely affects the normal hormonal status of military women.. Inadequate energy availability (a negative relationship between energy intake and activity level) changes the pulsatility of luteinizing hormone (LH) and the circulating levels of cortisol and thyroid hormones. Some of these hormonal changes are also associated with amenorrhea. The disruption of LH pulsatility may be caused by a decrease in hypothalamic GnRH pulsatility. The long-term consequence may be anovulation, decreased estrogen secretion, and increased bone resorption. Thus, caloric restriction may directly affect the accrual of peak bone mineral content. Disordered eating, although not well documented in the military, is associated with similar hormonal changes. Inadequate energy availability in military women may result from any of several practices including caloric restriction to attain or maintain body weight standards, disordered eating practices, or rapid increases in exercise levels (IOM, 1998).

Other conditions that induce estrogen deficiency may adversely affect bone health. Secondary amenorrhea may also arise from physical or emotional stress, therapy with GnRH agonists, and use of long-acting progestagens.

5. How can the military best ensure that the dietary intakes of active-duty women in training and throughout their military careers do not contribute to an increased incidence of stress fractures and osteoporosis?

Nutritional surveys of military women, as described in Table 1-6, reveal energy and calcium intakes in a number of different military facilities that are consistently lower than the Military Dietary Recommended Allowances (MRDAs). Thus, it is important that education programs for military women be aimed at meeting requirements for total energy needs as well as for nutrients supportive of optimal bone health. With consumption of appropriately high energy diets matched to meet the demands of physical training and fitness, higher intakes of calcium may be promoted. Obtaining the MRDAs from unfortified food stuffs has the advantage of providing intakes of other beneficial nutrients and food components.

Women should strive to maintain a stable body weight within weight-range and activity standards appropriate for their service and to refrain from episodes of repetitive dieting and weight loss so as not to disrupt normal hormonal rhythms (IOM, 1998). Stable body weight may be achieved through proper diet and participation in weight-bearing aerobic exercise activities, such as running, and walking. These measures will reduce the risk for stress fractures in the short term as well as for osteoporosis in the long term.

Eating fortified food products represents one method by which individuals can increase or maintain intakes without major changes in food habits (IOM, 1997). If women are unable to select foods and/or ration components to meet the MRDA for calcium, then appropriately formulated supplements could be considered.

CONCLUSIONS

Stress fractures incurred during military basic training have a significant impact on the physical fitness, training costs, and morbidity of military women. The initial fitness of recruits, both cardiorespiratory and musculoskeletal, appears to be the principal factor in the development of stress fractures during basic training.

As women enter military basic training, there may be insufficient time to achieve the aerobic fitness level required and the musculoskeletal adaptations necessary to avoid injury. Modifications to the basic training program that will promote achievement of the desired level of fitness and minimize training losses due to stress fractures could significantly influence training costs and retention of newly recruited military personnel. Training conditions that produce "optimum" levels of bone mass are important to the longer-term bone health of military women, especially during their later years when the incidence of osteoporosis normally increases.

Muscle mass, strength, and resistance to fatigue with cyclic loading play a critical role in development of stress fracture. Presentations at the workshop, *Reducing Stress Fracture in Physically Active Young Servicemembers,* indicated that certain training and/or fitness activities might predispose women to risk of stress fracture, especially in the pelvic region. These activities include dropping to the knees for push-ups, use of an unnatural gait or long strides during long marches, and use of incorrectly designed equipment such as footwear. Predisposing physical conditions, such as unequal leg length, have been shown to contribute to increased injury rates. In addition, the rate at which the intensity, frequency, and volume of loading occurs during training activities can increase risk for stress fractures.

Energy intake should be adequate to maintain weight during intensive physical fitness training. The requirements for adequate energy and nutrient intakes to meet the needs of the body at a moderate activity level are in the range of 2,000 to 2,800 kcal/d (AR 40-25, 1985). Nutritional modification of diets for incoming recruits are not effective in preventing stress fractures during the short term of basic training; however, modifications of diet may help to optimize overall bone health in the long term.

Currently, there is insufficient evidence to support the idea that calcium intake above the levels recommended for the general population will prevent stress fractures. In addition, data are too sparse to conclude that intense physical activity increases calcium requirements.

The requirement for military women to meet periodic military weight standards and physical fitness tests may induce inappropriate eating habits and or sudden changes in exercise training regimens, which may adversely affect bone health. Representative data are not available on the prevalence of disordered eating patterns among military women; however, dieting appears prevalent (IOM, 1998).

Conditions that induce estrogen deficiency from any cause (e.g., training regimen, diet, weight loss) may adversely affect the skeleton. It is likely that the maintenance of adequate energy intake is important in preventing the onset of secondary amenorrhea. Exogenous estrogen-progestogen hormones may positively affect peak bone mass reached in adulthood, which may be important for future fracture risks. Most of the evidence reviewed by the subcommittee indicated that there were no detrimental effects of the use of oral contraceptives on bone health. In contrast, long-acting progestogens may have a detrimental effect on bone mineral density (BMD), and therefore, their use should be discouraged at this time. Caution should be given regarding the long-term use of GnRH agonists to treat endometriosis because of the risk of inducing substantial bone loss.

Additionally, genetics and body mass, specifically skeletal muscle mass, are important determinants in the development of stress fractures. Reduced skeletal muscle mass has been associated with increased fatigability, whereas excessive skeletal muscle mass is associated with increased torque, contributing to fractures at specific anatomic sites. Moreover, except for rare instances where stress fractures result from an underlying metabolic bone disorder, there is currently no evidence that the risk of developing osteoporosis is increased in individuals who previously suffered a stress fracture.

RECOMMENDATIONS

Bone Mass and Bone Health

1. *The subcommittee recommends that bone measurements not be used routinely for screening recruits.* This is due to problems with the accuracy (both specificity and sensitivity) of ultrasound bone mineral content (BMC) measurements to predict stress fractures in military women and the fact that mean BMD measurements of athletes with fractures lie within the normal range. The subcommittee acknowledges that other current technologies such as dual energy x-ray absorptiometry (DXA), peripheral DXA (pDXA), quantitative computed tomography (QCT), and peripheral QCT (pQCT) may be useful for bone density assessment, but they cannot be used to screen for stress fractures.

2. *The subcommittee recommends that the military encourage behaviors that are consistent with optimizing bone health.* There are data suggesting an association between stress fracture and BMC coupled with the need to optimize bone mass for the prevention of osteoporosis,

Fitness and Training

3. *The subcommittee recommends that a more appropriate fitness standard be achieved by women prior to beginning basic training.* The military services should develop and/or adopt a gradual, stratified fitness program that best suits their individual training objectives. A fitness program for individuals who are not prepared to enter military basic training should be designed that starts women at a lower level of activity and gradually increases the activity level to prepare them for entry into basic training. The American College of Sports Medicine is one organization that publishes guidelines adequate for these purposes (ACSM, 1990). This prebasic training program should utilize training techniques similar to those employed in basic training. The overwhelming body of evidence reviewed by the BCNH subcommittee indicated that initial fitness level and the rate at which intensity of activity is increased are critical factors in placing women at risk for stress fractures. Excessive exercise and abrupt changes in training load should be avoided. Although this report addresses the

specific question of lowering the incidence of stress fractures in women, both men and women will benefit and have a lower incidence of stress fractures if they are required to meet an appropriate level of fitness before entering basic training.

4. *Consideration should be given to implementation of a standardized program of military basic training that encourages and focuses on gradual building of skeletal muscle mass with selected strength and endurance activities.* The military services should identify and modify activities that produce excessive skeletal muscle force on vulnerable bones; and establish (or modify) exercise habits in women that decrease selected stress fracture risks, similar to those programs and activities that have been proposed by the Naval Health Research Center (Almeida et al., 1997), the U.S. Air Force basic military training (BMT) group (Jaeger, 1996), and the Army's *Physical Fitness Training* manual (FM 21-20, 1992).

5. *The military should increase the emphasis on physical fitness programs for all active servicemembers.* This in turn will assist in the maintenance of weight, fat-free mass, and bone mass. More frequent fitness and body composition assessments would promote continuous adherence to weight and physical fitness programs and decrease high-risk behaviors that result from servicemembers' efforts to pass periodic performance and body composition tests.

6. *The subcommittee strongly suggests that the Department of Defense (DoD) consider joining with other federal agencies and programs to educate the young adult population about the importance of physical activity for health and well-being and to identify those individuals who might be at a high risk for stress fracture.* This role should be consistent with the DoD need to have a pool of recruits sufficiently fit for military training.

Reproductive Health and Bone Health

7. *The prevalence and underlying causes of oligomenorrhea and amenorrhea should be assessed in women undergoing basic training, advanced training, and active duty.* Because menstrual irregularities can result in bone loss, young women in the military should be provided with information about the associations among the menstrual cycle, estrogen sufficiency (including use of contraceptives), energy restriction, and bone health.

Energy Intake and Bone Health

8. *As recommended in its previous report (IOM, 1998), the BCNH subcommittee "reinforces the requirement for adequate energy and nutrient intakes to reflect the needs of the body at a moderate activity level (2,000–2,800 kcal/d).* Measures should be implemented to ensure that women's energy intakes are consistent and adequate to maintain weight during intensive physical fitness training. To ensure adequate nutrient intakes, female personnel must be educated on how to meet both energy and nutrient needs whether they are deployed and subsisting on operational rations or in garrison. (Many of these principles are outlined in the Army's *Physical Fitness Training* manual [FM 21-20, 1992].) This education is required to enable women to choose foods of higher nutrient density and to maintain a fitness program that allows for greater energy intake." The education program should be introduced within the training curriculum utilized during the Delayed Entry Program to emphasize the importance and relationship of energy and nutrient

balance to weight control. "The committee reinforces the recent efforts of the Army to provide complete nutritional labeling of all ration components and to include information to enable identification of nutrient-dense components that would help women meet the MRDAs at their usual energy intake. The committee also supports efforts to create ration supplements that would satisfy requirements that may not be readily met through the usual intake of rations. The committee recommends nutritional labeling of all dining hall menu items and provision of food selection guidelines to women in garrison" (IOM, 1998, p. 162).

9. *Aggressive education programs should be aimed at women to help them identify and select appropriate foods, including calcium-fortified food products, thus increasing the number of women meeting their requirement for nutrients essential to bone health.* The recommended Adequate Intake for calcium in women aged 19 through 30 years is set at 1,000 mg/d (NRC, 1997), which is consistent with the current MRDAs of 800 to 1,200 mg/d. However, calcium intakes in military women are reported to meet only 75 percent of the MRDA, principally because women often do not consume their full ration components. Data on the intake of vitamin D are not routinely captured in military surveys. Nevertheless, results from military intake studies strongly suggest that because of the lower level of consumption of operational rations and dining hall meals that are based on a 3,600 kcal diet plan, active-duty women are at risk for inadequate intake of several nutrients, particularly calcium. To ensure adequate energy and nutrient intake, some modifications of operational rations may be needed to increase the nutrient density. If adequate intakes of calcium are not being met from operational (field) rations or in garrison, and if nutrition education and counseling sessions fail to promote increased intakes, the use of calcium-fortified products is essential. Calcium supplements should be recommended under appropriate guidance by the military to meet women's special needs.

RECOMMENDATIONS FOR FUTURE RESEARCH

1. A minimal fitness standard is currently used to allow women to enter basic training. Research is needed to define the appropriate fitness level required for women to enter the military and participate in basic training without incurring an increased risk of stress fractures.

2. Efforts should be made to compile data from all military services on initial fitness levels of recruits by age, gender, and race/ethnicity.

3. As recommended in the *Report on Injuries in the Military: The Hidden Epidemic* (AFEB, 1996), further study is needed to determine the types of activities that may predispose women to stress fractures, especially in the pelvic region and upper leg. Steps should be taken to modify activities in basic training to lower risk.

4. The subcommittee recommends that the military services collect stress fracture incidence statistics by age, gender, race/ethnicity, and skeletal site, using a gender-independent, standardized definition and collecting data during a comparable time frame from all military services during both the basic-training and post training periods. Although no uniform outpatient surveillance system exists throughout the DoD, the Naval Health Research Center (Almeida et al., 1997) has developed a software application program for the purpose of supporting epidemiological research in musculoskeletal injuries. This may provide the basis for a model for the collection of injury-related data.

5. Because the military primarily recruits from a population that is accruing its peak bone mass, the BCNH subcommittee recommends that research efforts should contribute to identifying those factors, such as diet, lifestyle, and ethnicity, that may contribute to achieving peak bone mass, as well as components of military programs that may interfere with this process. The *Report on Injuries in the Military: The Hidden Epidemic* (AFEB, 1996) similarly recommends the identification and surveillance of those risk factors contributing to stress fracture injuries.

6. Efforts should be made to investigate more fully the now-preliminary linkages between low skeletal muscle mass, particularly in women, and stress fracture risk. Investigators should attempt to determine if this injury risk is a result of low skeletal muscle mass *per se* or a manifestation of inappropriately designed or enforced training programs.

7. Most of the evidence reviewed by the BCNH subcommittee indicated no detrimental effects on bone health from the use of oral contraceptives. However, the subcommittee recommends that future research is needed on the effects of implant or injectable contraceptives, such as Depo-Provera, on BMD and bone strength. Chemical formulation, dosage, and route of administration require further investigation.

8. Research is needed to assess the effect of military women's dietary energy status on the secretion of hormones that affect bone health, particularly in situations of high metabolic stress. Little is known about predisposing factors that alter the menstrual cycle.

9. The military should continue to gather dietary intake data and evidence concerning calcium intakes throughout a soldier's career as training programs, food choices, and food supply change over time.

10. Based on preliminary data from athletes, loss of calcium in sweat due to physical exertion during training as a potential pathophysiological factor on the development of stress fracture needs to be investigated. These preliminary data raise a broader question about the impact of high levels of activity on calcium requirement.

11. More research is needed that evaluates existing technologies of assessing risk of stress fracture, including ultrasound, central and peripheral DXA and central and peripheral QCT. Ultimately the cost-benefit analysis of all techniques will have to be assessed for specific uses and populations within the military.

12. The DoD should support the development of mechanical models that link skeletal muscle mass, force/torque, and bone stress in humans. As part of this process, efforts should be made to improve existing *in vivo* methods of quantifying components of these models, including mechanical loads and skeletal muscle mass.

Bibliography

ACSM (American College of Sports Medicine). 1997. ACSM position stand. The female athlete triad. Med. Sci. Sports. Exerc. 29:i–ix.

AFEB (Armed Forces Epidemiological Board) 1996. Injuries in the military: a hidden epidemic. Report 29 HA 4844 97.Falls Church, Virg.: Armed Forces Epidemiologic Board.

Alfredson, H., P. Nordstrom, and R. Lorentzon. 1996. Total and regional bone mass in female soccer players. Calcif. Tissue Int. 59:438–442.

Almeida, S.A., K.M. Williams, R.A. Shaffer, J.T. Luz, E. Badong, and S.K. Brodine. 1997. A physical training program to reduce musculoskeletal injuries in U.S. Marine Corps recruits. Technical Document No. 97-2B. San Diego, Calif.: Naval Health Research Center.

AR (Army Regulation) 40-25. 1985. *See* U.S. Departments of the Army, the Navy, and the Air Force, 1985.

Aurbach, G.D., S.J. Marx, and A.M. Spiegel. 1992. Parathyroid hormone, calcitonin, and the calciferols. Pp. 1397–1476 in Williams Textbook of Endocrinology, J.E. Wilson and D.W. Foster, eds. Philadelphia: W.B. Saunders Company.

Baren, D., A. Sorensen, J. Grimes, R. Lew, A. Karellas, B. Johnson, J. Roche. 1990. Dietary modification with dairy products for preventing vertebral bone loss in premenopausal women; a three-year prospective study. J. Clin. Endocrinol. Metab. 70(1):264-270.

Bates et al. 1983. An assessment of subject variability, subject-shoe interaction, and the evaluation of running shoes using ground reaction force data. J. Biomech. 16(3):181–91.

Beals, K.A., and M.M. Manore. 1994. The prevalence and consequence of subclinical eating disorders in female athletes. Int. J. Sports Nutr. 4:175–195.

Beck, T.J. 1997. Structural indices of stress fracture susceptibility in female military recruits. Presentation at the workshop on Reducing Stress Fracture in Physically Active Young Servicemembers, December 10, Washington, D.C.

Beck, T., C. Ruff, F. Mourtada, R. Shaffer, K. Maxwell-Williams, G. Kao, D. Sartoris, and S. Brodine. 1996. DXA derived structural geometry for stress fracture prediction in male U.S. Marine Corps recruits. J. Bone Miner. Res. 11:645–653.

Bell, N.S., T.W. Mangione, D. Hemenway, P.J. Amoroso, and B.H. Jones. Submitted. High injury rates among female Army trainees: A function of gender?

Bell, 1994. Injury etiology and prevention: selected topics. Doctoral thesis, Harvard School of Public Health.

Bennell, K.L., S.A. Malcolm, S.A. Thomas, S.J. Reid, P.D. Brukner, P.R. Ebeling, and J.D. Wark. 1996. Risk factors for stress fracture in track and field athletes. Am. J. Sports Med. 24:810–818.

Bentley, W. 1978. Policy guidance for organized physical training. Memorandum for the US Army, Europe, and 7th Army, October 30, 1978.

Bilanin, J., M. Blanchard, and E. Russek-Cohen. 1989. Lower vertebral bone density in male long distance runners. Med. Sci. Sports Exerc. 21:66–70.

Boivin, G., C. Anthoine-Terrier, and K.J. Obrant. 1990. Transmission electron microscopy of bone tissue. A review. J. Bone Miner. Res. 5 S1:S185–9.

Bouxsein, M.L., and R. Marcus. 1994. Overview of exercise and bone mass. Rheum. Dis. Clin. North Am. 20:787–802.

Brudvig, T.J., T.D. Grudger, and L. Obermeyer. 1983. Stress fractures in 295 trainees: A 1-year study of incidence related to age, sex, and race. Mil. Med. 148:666–667.

Brukner, P. 1997. Stress fracture among physically active women in the general population. Presentation at the workshop on Reducing Stress Fracture in Physically Active Young Servicemembers, December 10, Washington, D.C.

Brukner, P., and K. Bennell. 1997. Stress fractures in females athletes. Diagnosis, management and rehabilitation. Sports Med. 24(6):419–429.

Buckwalter, J.A., M.J. Glimcher, R.R. Cooper, and R Recker. 1996. Bone biology. I: Structure, blood supply, cells, matrix, and mineralization. Instr. Course Lect. 45:371–86..

Bullen, B.A., G.S. Skrinar, I.Z. Beitins, G. Von Mering, B.A. Trunbull, and J.W. MacArthur. 1985. Induction of menstrual disorders by strenuous exercise in untrained women. N. Engl. J. Med. 312:1349–1353.

Burr, D.B. 1997. Muscle strength, bone mass, and age-related bone loss. J. Bone Miner. Res. 12:1547–1551.

Burrows, H.J. 1956. Fatigue infraction of the middle of the tibia in ballet dancers. J. Bone Joint Surg. 38B:83–94.

Canham, M.L., M.A. McFerren, and B.H. Jones. 1996. The association of injury with physical fitness among men and women in gender integrated basic combat training units. MSMR 2(4):8–10.

Cavanagh, P.R. 1980. The Running Shoe Book. Mountain View, Calif.: Anderson World.

Cavanagh, P.R., and M.A. Lafortune. 1980. Ground reaction forces in distance running. J. Biomech. 13(5):397–406.

Charles, P., F.T. Jensen, L. Mosekilde, and H.H. Hansen. 1983. Calcium metabolism evaluated at ^{47}Cs kinetics: estimation of dermal calcium loss. Clin. Sci. 65(4):415–422.

Charles, P., E.F. Eriksen, C. Hashing, K. Sondergard, and L. Mosekilde. 1991. Dermal, intestinal, and renal obligatory losses of calcium: Relation to skeletal calcium loss. Am. J. Clin. Nutr. 54(suppl):266S–272S·

Chen, Z., T.G. Lohman, W.A. Stini, C. Rittenbaugh, and M. Aickin. 1997. Fat or lean tissue mass: Which one is the major determinant of bone mineral mass in healthy post-menopausal women. J. Bone Miner. Res. 12:144–151.

Clapp III, J.F., and K.D. Little. 1995. The interaction between regular exercise and selected aspects of women's health. Am. J. Obstet. Gynecol. 173:2–9.

Clement, D.B., J.E. Taunton, G.W. Smart, et al. 1981. A survey of overuse running injuries. Phys. Sportsmed. 9:47–58.

Compston, J., M. Laskey, P. Croucher, A. Coxon, and S. Kreitzman. 1992. Effect of diet-induced weight loss on total body bone mass. Clin. Sci. 82:429–432.

Conover, C.A. 1996. The role of insulin-like growth factors and binding proteins in bone cell biology. Pp. 607–618 in Principles of Bone Biology, J.P. Bilezikian, L.G. Raisz, and G.A. Rodan, eds. San Diego, Calif.: Academic Press.

Cowin, S.C., L. Moss-Salentijn, and M.L. Moss. 1991. Candidates for the mechnosensory system in bone. J. Biomech. Eng. 113(2):191–7.

Cumming, D.C. 1996. Exercise-associated amenorrhea, low bone density, and estrogen replacement therapy. Arch. Intern. Med. 156:2193–2195.

Cundy, T., M. Evans, and H. Roberts. 1991. Bone density in women receiving depot medroxy progesterone acetate for contraception. Br. Med. J. 303:13–16.

Dawson-Hughes, B., G.E. Dallal, E.A. Krall, L. Sadowski, N. Sahyoun, and S. Tannenbaum. 1990. A controlled trial of the effect of calcium supplementation on bone density in postmenopausal women. N. Engl. J. Med. 323(13):878-883.

DeCherney, A. 1996. Bone-sparing properties of oral contraceptives. Am. J. Obstet. Gynecol. 174:15–20.

De Souza, M.J., B.E. Miller, L.C. Sequenzia, A.A. Luciano, S. Ulreuch, S. Stier, K. Prestwood, and B.L. Lasley. 1997. Bone health is not affected by luteal phase abnormalities and decreased ovarian progesterone production in female runners. 82(9):2867–2876.

Deporte, E., and B. Van Gheluwe. 1989. Ground reaction forces in elite high jumping. ISB XII. Los Angeles: International Congress of Biomechanics·

Dickinson, J.A., Cook S.D., Leinhardt, T.M. 1985. The measurement of shock waves following heel strike while running. J. Biomech. 18:415–422.

Doyle, F., J. Brown, and C. Lachance. 1970. Relation between bone mass and muscle weight. Lancet 1(7643):391–393.

Drake III, A.J. 1996. Characteristics of female midshipmen: 1992 to 1996. Presentation at the workshop on Assessing Readiness in Military Women: The Relationship to Nutrition. September 9–10, Irvine, Calif. [*see* IOM, 1998].

Drinkwater, B.L., K. Nilson, C.H. Chesnut, W.J. Bremner, S. Shainholtz, and M.B. Southworth. 1984. Bone mineral content of amenorrheic and eumenorrheic athletes. N. Engl. J. Med. 311:277–281.

Dueck, C.A., K.S. Matt, M.M. Manore, and J.S. Skinner. 1996. Treatment of athletic amenorrhea with a diet and training intervention program. Int. J. Sports Nutr. 6:24–40.

Dufek, J.S., and B.T. Bates. 1991. Biomechanical factors associated with injury during landing in jump sports. Sports Med. 12(5):326–337.

Ellis, K.J., and S.H. Cohn. 1975. Correlation between skeletal calcium mass and muscle mass in man. J. Appl. Physiol. 38(3):455–60.

Engh, C.A., R.A. Robinson, and J. Milgram. 1970. Stress fractures in children. J. Trauma 10(7):532–541.

Enzelsberger, H., M. Metka, and G. Heytmanek. 1988. Influence of oral contraceptive use on bone density in climacteric women. Maturitas 9:375–378.

Etherington, J., P.A. Harris, D. Nandra, D.J. Hart, R.L. Wolman, D.V. Doyle, and T.D. Spector. 1996. The effect of weight-bearing exercise on bone mineral density: A study of female ex-elite athletes and the general population. J. Bone Miner. Res. 11:1333–1338.

FM (Field Manual) 21-20. *See* U.S. Department of the Army, 1992.

Frederick, E.C. and J.L. Hagy. 1986. Factors affecting peak vertical ground reaction forces in running. Int. J. Sport Biomechanics. 2:41-49.

Frederick, E.C., T.E. Clarke. 1981. Consequences of scaling on impact loading in running. Medicine and Science in Sport and Exercise 3(13):96.

Fredericson, M. 1996. Common injuries in runners. Diagnosis, rehabilitation and prevention. Sports Med. 21(1):49–72.

Garner, D.M., and M.P. Olmstead. 1991. The Eating Disorders Inventory 2. Odessa, Fla.: Psychological Assessment Resources, Inc.

Garnero, P., E. Sornay-Rendu, and P.D. Delmas. 1995. Decreased bone turnover in oral contraceptive users. Bone 16:499–503.

Ghiron, L.J., J.L. Thompson, L. Holloway, R.L. Hintz, G.E. Butterfield, A.R. Hoffman and R. Marcus. 1995. Effects of recombinant insulin-like growth factor-I and growth hormone on bone turnover in elderly women. J. Bone Miner. Res. 10:1844–1852.

Girasole, G., R.L. Jilka, G. Passeri, S. Boswell, G. Boder, D.C. Williams, and S.C. Manolagas. 1992. 17 beta-estradiol inhibits interleukin-6 production by bone marrow-derived stromal cells and osteoblasts in vitro: a potential mechanism for the antiosteoporotic effect of estrogens. J. Clin. Invest. 89(3):883–91.

Gluer, C.C., S.R. Cummings, D.C. Bauer, K. Stone, A. Pressman, A. Mathur, and H.K. Genant. 1996. Osteoporosis: Association of recent fractures with quantitative U.S. findings. Radiology 199:725–732.

Goldsmith, N.F., and J.O. Johnston. 1975. Bone mineral effects of oral contraceptives, pregnancy, and lactation. J. Bone Joint Surg. 57:657–668.

Graham, J.D., and C.L. Clarke. 1997. Physiological action of progesterone in target tissues. Endocr. Rev. 18:502–519.

Hall, M.L., J. Heavens, I.D. Cullum, and P.J. Ell. 1990. The range of bone density in normal British women. Br. J. Radiol. 63:266–269.

Hamill, J., B.T. Bates, K.M. Knutzen, and J.A. Sawhill. 1983. Variations in ground reaction force parameters at different running speeds. Human Movement Science. 2:47–56.

Hamill, C.L., T.E. Clarke, E.C. Frederick, L.J. Goodyear, and E.T. Howley. 1984. Effects of grade running on kinematics and impact force. Med. Sci. Sports Exerc. 16:185.

Heaney, R.P. 1996. Bone mass, nutrition, and other lifestyle factors. Nutr. Rev. 54:S3–S10

Henderson, R.C., G.J. Kemp, and E.R. Campion. 1992. Residual bone mineral density and muscle strength after fractures of the tibia or femur in children. J. Bone Joint Surg. 74:211–218.

Hergenroeder, A.C. 1995. Bone mineralization, hypothalamic amenorrhea, and sex steroid therapy in female adolescents and young adults. J. Pediatr. 126:683–689.

Hergenroeder, A.C., E.O. Smith, R. Shypailo, L.A. Jones, W.J. Klish, and K. Ellis. 1997. Bone mineral changes in young women with hypothalamic amenorrhea treated with oral contraceptives, medroxyprogesterone, or placebo over 12 months. Am. J. Obstet. Gynecol. 176:1017–1025.

Honkanen, R., E.M. Alhava, S. Saarikoski, and M. Tuppurainen. 1991. Osteoporosis risk factors in perimenopausal women. Calcif. Tissue Int. 49:S74–S75.

Hourani, L.L. 1996. Health and nutrition profile of women in the Navy. Presentation at the workshop on Assessing Readiness in Military Women: The Relationship to Nutrition. September 9–10, Irvine, Calif. [*see* IOM, 1998].

Hreshchyshyn, M.M., A. Hopkins, S. Zylstra, and M. Anbar. 1988. Associations of parity, breast-feeding, and birth control pills with lumbar spine and femoral neck bone densities. Am. J. Obstet. Gynecol. 159:318–322.

IOM (Institute of Medicine). 1992. Body Composition and Physical Performance, Applications for the Military Services, B.M. Marriott and J. Grumstrup-Scott, eds. Committee on Military Nutrition Research, Food and Nutrition Board. Washington, D.C.: National Academy Press.

IOM (Institute of Medicine) 1997. Dietary Reference Intakes for Calcium, Phosphorus, Magnesium, Vitamin D, and Fluoride [prepublication copy]. Standing Committee on the Scientific Evaluation of Dietary Reference Intakes, Food and Nutrition Board. Washington, D.C.: National Academy Press.

IOM (Institute of Medicine). 1998. Assessing Readiness in Military Women: The Relationship to Body Composition, Nutrition, and Health. Committee on Body Composition, Nutrition, and Health of Military Women, Committee on Military Nutrition Research, Food and Nutrition Board. Washington, D.C.: National Academy Press.

Jaeger, B.R. et al., 1996. USAF recruit fitness study. Brooks AFB, Tex.: Detachment 1, Human Systems Center, Office for Prevention and Health Services Assessment.

James, S.L. et al., 1978. Injuries to runners. Am. J. Sports. Med. 6(2):40-50.

Jensen, L.B., F. Quaade, and O.H. Sorensen. 1994. Bone loss accompanying voluntary weight loss in obese humans. J. Bone Miner. Res. 9:459–463.

Johnell, O., A. Rausing, B. Wendeberg, and N. Westlin. 1982. Morphological bone changes in shin splints. Clin. Orthop. 167:180–184.

Johnson, L.C., H.T. Stradford, R.W. Geis, J.R. Dineen, and E. Kerley. 1963. Histogenesis of stress fractures. J. Bone Joint Surg. 45A:1542.

Johnson, A.W., C.B. Weiss, and D.L. Wheeler. 1994. Stress fracture of the femoral shaft in athletes—more common than expected. A new clinical test. Am. J. Sports Med. 22:248–256.

Jones, B.H. 1983. Overuse injuries of the lower extremities associated with marching, jogging, and running: A review. Milit. Med. 148:783–787.

Jones, B.H., J.M. Harris, T.N. Vinh, and C. Rubin. 1989. Exercise-induced stress fractures and stress reactions of bone: Epidemiology, etiology, and classification. Exerc. Sport Sci. Rev. 17:379–422.

Kannus, P., M. Jarvinen, H. Sievanen, P. Oja, and I. Vuori. 1994. Osteoporosis in men with a history of tibial fracture. J. Bone Miner. Res. 9:423–429.

Kelly, P.J., and J.A. Eisman. 1992. Osteoporosis: Genetic effects on bone turnover and bone density. Ann. Med. 25:100–101.

Kelsey, J.L., W.S. Browner, D.G. Seeley, M.C. Nevitt, and S.R. Cummings. 1992. Risk factors for fractures of the distal forearm and proximal humerus. Am. J. Epidemiol. 135:477–489.

King, N., K.E. Fridlund and E.W. Askew. 1993. Nutrition Issues in Military Women. J. Am. Coll. Nutr. 12:344–348.

Kiratli, B.J. 1996. Immobilization osteopenia. Pp. 833–853 in Osteoporosis, R. Marcus, D. Feldman, and J. Kelsey, eds. San Diego, Calif.: Academic Press.

Kleerekoper, M., R.S. Brienza, and L.R. Schultz. 1991. Oral contraceptive use may protect against low bone mass: Henry Ford Hospital Osteoporosis Cooperative Research Group. Arch. Intern. Med. 151:1971–1976.

Kleerekoper, M. 1997. Effect of Modulators of Bone Turnover on Changes in Markers of Bone Turnover. Presentation at the workshop on Reducing Stress Fracture in Physically Active Young Servicemembers, December 10, Washington, D.C.

Klesges, R.C., K.D. Ward, M.L. Shelton, W.B. Applegate, E.D. Cantler, G.M. Palmieri, K. Harmon, and J. Davis. 1996. Changes in bone mineral content in male athletes: Mechanisms of action and intervention effects. J. Am. Med. Assoc. 276:226–230.

Klibanski, A., B.M.K. Biller, D.A. Schoenfeld, D.B. Herzog, and V.C. Saxe. 1995. The effects of estrogen administration on trabecular bone loss in young women with anorexia nervosa. J. Clin. Endocrinol. Metab. 80:898–904.

Klicka, M.V., D.E. Sherman, N. King, K.E. Friedl, and E.W. Askew. 1993. Nutritional assessment of U.S. Military Academy cadets at West Point: Part 2. Assessment of nutritional intake. Technical Report No. T94-1. Natick, Mass.: U.S. Army Research Institute of Environmental Medicine.

Knapik, J., and N. Henderson. 1997. Injury incidence in soldiers attending Medical Specialist (MOS91B) AIT, Fort Sam Houston, Texas. MSMR 3:10–12.

Kowal, D.M. 1980. Nature and causes of injuries in women resulting from an endurance training program. Am. J. Sports Med. 8(4):265–269.

Krall, E.A., and B. Dawson-Hughes. 1993. Heritable and life-style determinants of bone mineral density. J. Bone Miner. Res. 8:1–9.

Kritz-Silverstein, D., and E. Barrett-Connor. 1993. Bone mineral density in postmenopausal women as determined by prior oral contraceptive use. Am. J. Publ. Health 83:100–102.

Kurzer, M.S., and D.H. Calloway. 1986. Effects of energy deprivation on sex hormone patterns in healthy menstruating women. Am. J. Physiol. 251(4 pt. 1):E483–488.

Laitinen, K., and M. Valimaki. 1991. Alcohol and bone. Calcif. Tissue Int. 49:S70–S73.

Lauder, T. 1997. The female athlete triad: Prevalence in military women. ADA330021. Tacoma, Wash.: Madigan Army Medical Center.

Laughlin, G.A., C.E. Dominguez, A.J. Morales, and S.S.C. Yen. 1994. Alterations of insulin/glucose and the GH-IGF-IGFBP system during the 25h metabolic clock in cycling and amenorrheic athletes [abstract 842]. P. 411 in Proceedings of the 76th Annual Meeting of the Endocrine Society.

Law, M.R., and A.K. Hackshaw. 1997. A meta-analysis of cigarette smoking, bone mineral density, and risk of hip fracture: Recognition of a major effect. Br. Med. J. 315:841–846.

Li, G., S.D. Zhang, G. Cheng, H. Chen, and A.M. Wang. 1985. Radiographic and histologic analyses of stress fracture in rabbit tibias. Am. J. Sports Med. 13(5):285–94.

Light, L.H., G.E. McLellan, and L. Klenerman. 1980. Skeletal transients on heel strike in normal walking with different footwear. J. Biomech. 13:477–480.

Lindsay, R., J. Tohme, and B. Kanders. 1986. The effect of oral contraceptive use on vertebral bone mass in pre- and postmenopausal women. Contraception 34:333–340.

Loucks, A.B. 1989. Athletics and menstrual dysfunction in young women. Pp. 513–538 in Perspectives in Exercise Science and Sports Medicine, vol. 2: Youth, Exercise, and Sport, G.V. Gisolfi and D.R. Lamb, eds. Indianapolis: Benchmark Press.

Loucks, A.B. 1996. The reproductive system. Pp. 41–66 in Perspectives in Exercise Science and Sports Medicine, vol. 9: Exercise and the Female—A Life-Span Approach, O. Bar-Or, D. Lamb, and P. Clarkson, eds. Carmel, Ind.: Cooper Publishing Group.

Loucks, A.B., and R. Callister. 1993. Induction and prevention of low T3-syndrome in exercising women. Am. J. Physiol. 264:R924–R930.

Loucks, A.B., and E.M. Heath. 1994. Induction of low T3-syndrome in exercising women occurs at a threshold of energy availability. Am. J. Physiol. 266:R817–R823.

Loucks, A.B., G.L. Laughlin, J.F. Mortola, L. Girton, J.C. Nelson, and S.S.C. 1992. Yen. Hypothalamic-pituitary-thyroidal function in eumenorrheic and amenorrheic athletes. J. Clin. Endocrinol. Metab. 75:514–518.

Lu, P.W., J.N. Briody, G.D. Ogle, K. Morley, I.R. Humphries, J. Allen, R. Howman-Giles, D. Sillence, and C.T. Cowell. 1994. Bone mineral density of total body, spine, and femoral neck in children and young adults: A cross-sectional and longitudinal study. J. Bone Miner. Res. 9:1451–1458.

Lukert, B.P., and B.E. Kream. 1996. Clinical and basic aspects of glucocorticoid action in bone. Pp. 533–548 in Principles of Bone Biology, J.P. Bilezikian, L.G. Raisz, and G.A. Rodan, eds. San Diego, Calif.: Academic Press, Inc.

Marcus, R. 1991. Understanding osteoporosis. West J. Med. 155(1):53-60

Marcus, R. 1996. Mechanisms of exercise. Effects on bone. Pp. 1135–1146 in Principles of Bone Biology, J.P. Bilezikian, L.G. Raisz, and G.A. Rodan, eds. San Diego, Calif.: Academic Press, Inc.

Marcus, R., C. Cann, P. Madvig, J. Minkoff, M. Goddard, M. Bayer, M. Martin, L. Guadiani, W. Haskell, and H. Genant. 1985. Menstrual function and bone mass in elite women distance runners. Ann. Int. Med. 102:158–163.

Margolis, R.N., E. Canalis, and N.C. Partridge. 1996. Invited review of a workshop. Anabolic hormones in bone: Basic research and therapeutic potential. J. Clin. Endocrinol. Metab. 81:872–877.

Marks Jr., S.C., and S.N. Popoff. 1988. Bone cell biology: The regulation of development, structure, and function in the skeleton. Am. J. Anat. 183(1):1–44.

Marshall, D., O. Johnell, and H. Wedel. 1996. Meta-analysis of how well measures of bone mineral density predict occurrence of osteoporotic fractures. Br. Med. J. 312:1254–1259.

Marti, B., J.P. Vader, C.. Minder et al. 1988. On the epidemiology of running injuries: The 1984 Bern Grand-Prix study. Am. J. Sports Med. 16:285–294.

Martin, R.B.. 1991. On the significance of remodeling space and activation rate changes in bone remodeling. Bone. 12(6):391–400.

Martin, D.B., and R.B. Burr. 1989. Errors in bone remodeling: Toward a unified theory of metabolic bone disease. Am. J. Anat. 186(2):186–216.

Matheson, G.O., D.B. Clement, D.C. McKenzie, J.E. Taunton, D.R. Lloyd-Smith, and J.G. Macintyre. 1987a. Scintigraphic uptake of 99mTc at non-painful sites in athletes with stress fractures: The concept of bone strain. Sports Med. 4:65–75.

Matheson, G.O., D.B. Clement, D.C. McKenzie, J.E. Taunton, D.R. Lloyd-Smith, and J.G. Macintyre. 1987b. Stress fractures in athletes: A study of 320 cases. Am. J. Sports Med. 15(1):46–58.

Mazes, R.B., and H.S. Barden. 1991. Bone density in premenopausal women: Effects of age, dietary intake, physical activity, smoking, and birth control pills. Am. J. Clin. Nutr. 53:132–142.

McDermott. 1996. Assessment of dietary calcium intake, physical activity, and habits affecting skeletal health among premenopausal military women (protocol #9). ADA326553. Fitzsimmons Army Medical Center.

McNitt-Gray, J.L.. 1993. Kinetics of the lower extremities during drop landings from three heights. J. Biomech. 26(9):1037–1046.

Meghji, S. 1992. Bone remodelling. Br. Dent. J. 172(6):235–42.

Mehta, S. 1993. Bone loss, contraception, and lactation. Acta. Obstet. Gynecol. Scand. 72:148–156.

Michael, R.H., and L.E. Holder. 1985. The soleus syndrome. A cause of medial tibial stress (shin splints). Am. J. Sports Med. 13(2):87–94.

Montgomery, L.C., F.R. Nelson, J.P. Norton, and P.A. Deuster. 1989. Orthopedic history and examination in the etiology of overuse injuries. Med. Sci. Sports Exerc. 21:237–243.

Mori, S., and D.B. Burr. 1993. Increased intracortical remodeling following fatigue damage. Bone 14(2):103–109.

Moro, M., A.T. Hecker, M.L. Bouxsein, and E.R. Myers. 1995. Failure load of thoracic vertebrae correlates with lumbar bone mineral density measured by DXA. Calcif. Tissue Int. 56:206–209.

MSMR. 1997. Spontaneous fractures of the femur, active-duty soldiers. 3:2–9.

Mulligan, K., and G.E. Butterfield. 1990. Discrepancies between energy intake and expenditure in physically active women. Br. J. Nutr. 64:23–36.

Murphy, S., K. Khaw, and J.E. Compston. 1993. Lack of relationship between hip and spine bone mineral density and oral contraceptive use. Eur. J. Clin. Invest. 23:108–111.

Myburgh, K.H., J. Hutchins, A.B. Fataar, S.F. Hough, and T.D. Noakes. 1990. Low bone density is an etiologic factor for stress fractures in athletes. Ann. Intern. Med. 113:754–759.

Naessen, T., S. Olsson, and J. Gudmundson. 1995. Differential effects on bone density of progestogen-only methods for contraception in premenopausal women. Contraception 52:35–39.

Nigg, B.M., and B. Segesser. 1988. The influence of playing surfaces on the load on the locomotor system and on football and tennis injuries. Sports Med. 5(6):375–385.

Nigg, B.M., H.A. Bahlsen, S.M. Luethi, and S. Stokes. 1987. The influence of running velocity and midsole hardness on external impact forces in heel-toe running. 20(10):951–9.

Nike, Inc. 1987. Common running injuries. Sports Res. Rev. March 1-4.

Notelovitz, M., D. Martin, and R. Tesar. 1991. Estrogen therapy and variable-resistance weight training increase bone mineral in surgically menopausal women. J. Bone Miner. Res. 6:583–590.

NRC (National Research Council). 1989. Diet and Health: Implications for Reducing Chronic Disease Risk. Committee on Diet and Health, Food and Nutrition Board, Commission on Life Sciences. Washington, D.C.: National Academy Press.

Orth, D.N., W.J. Kovacs, and R. DeBold. 1992. The adrenal cortex. Pp. 489–619 in Williams Textbook of Endocrinology, J.D. Wilson and D.W. Foster, eds. Philadelphia: W.B. Saunders.

O'Toole, M.L. 1992. Prevention and treatment of injuries to runners. Med. Sci. Sports Exerc. 24(9 Suppl):S360–3.

Pagliano, J. and D. Jackson. 1980. The ultimate study of running injuries. Runner's World. 15:42–50.

Parfitt, A.M. 1988. Bone remodeling. Henry Ford Hospital Med. J.36(3):143–4.

Peacock, M. 1991. Calcium absorption efficiency and calcium requirements in children and adolescents. Am. J. Clin. Nutr. 54:261S–5S.

Peck, W.A., and W.L. Woods. 1988. The cells of bone.. In: B.L. R, ed. Osteoporosis: etiology, diagnosis, and management. New York: Raven Press.

Pilbeam, C.C., J.R. Harrison, and L.G. Raisz. 1996. Prostaglandins and bone metabolism. Pp. 715–728 in Principles of Bone Biology, J.P. Bilezikian, L.G. Raisz, and G.A. Rodan, eds. San Diego, Calif.: Academic Press, Inc.

Ramey, M.R., K.R. Williams. 1985. Ground Reaction Forces in the Triple Jump. International Journal of Sport Biomechanics. 1:233-239.

Ramsdale, S.J., and E.J. Bassey. 1994. Changes in bone mineral density associated with dietary-induced loss of body mass in young women. Clin. Sci. 87:343–348.

Rebuffe-Scrive, M., J. Eldh, and L.O. Bjorntorp. 1986. Metabolism of mammary, abdominal, and femoral adipocytes in women before and after menopause. Metabolism. 35:79–797.

Recker, R.R., K.M. Davies, and S.M. Hinders. 1992. Bone gain in young adult women. J. Am. Med. Assoc. 268:2403–2408.

Reinker, K.A., and S. Ozburne. 1979. A comparison of male and female orthopedic pathology in basic training. Mil. Med. 144:532–536.

Rencken, M.L., C.H. Chesnut 3rd, and B.L. Drinkwater 1996. Bone density at multiple skeletal sites in amenorrheic athletes. JAMA. 276(3)238–40.

Report of the Federal Advisory Committee on Gender-Integrated Training and Related Issues, to the Secretary of Defense, December 1997.

Riis, B.J., J.S. Christiansen, and J.S. Johansen. 1990. Is it possible to prevent bone loss in young women treated with luteinizing hormone-releasing hormone agonists? J. Clin. Endocrinol. Metab. 70:920–924.

Roberts, S.M., and E.C. Vogt. 1939. Pseudofracture of the tibia. J. Bone Joint Surg. 21:891–898.

Rosen, C.J. 1997. Insulin-like growth factor-I and parathyroid hormone: Potential new therapeutic agents for the treatment of osteoporosis. Exp. Opin. Invest. Drugs 6:1193–1198.

Rosen, C.J., H.P. Dimai, D. Vereault, L.R. Donahue, W.G. Beamer, J. Farley, S. Linkhart, T. Linkhart, S. Mohan, and D.J. Baylink. 1997. Circulating and skeletal insulin-like growth factor-I (IGF-I) concentrations in two inbred strains of mice with different bone mineral densities. Bone 21:217–223.

Sambrook, P., P. Kelly, and J. Eisman. 1993. Bone mass and aging. Baillière's Clin. Rheumatol. 7:445–457.

Sambrook, P.N., P.J. Kelly, C.P. White, N.A. Morrison, and J.A. Eisman. 1996. Genetic determinants of bone mass. Pages 477–482 in Osteoporosis, R. Marcus, D. Feldman, and J. Kelsey, eds. San Diego, Calif.: Academic Press.

Schmidt, A., S. Harada, and G.A. Rodan. 1996. Anabolic steroid effects on bone in women. Pp. 1125–1134 in Principles of Bone Biology, J.P. Bilezikian, L.G. Raisz, and G.A. Rodan, eds. San Diego, Calif.: Academic Press, Inc.

Schmitz, M. 1995. Confirmed: Smoking delays bone union. Orthop. Today 15:1, 23.

Schwellnus, M.P., and G. Jordaan. 1992. Does calcium supplementation prevent bone stress injuries? A clinical trial. Int. J. Sport Nutr. 2:165–174.

Shaffer, R.A. 1997. Physical training interventions to reduce stress fracture incidence in Navy and Marine Corps recruit training. Presentation at the workshop on Reducing Stress Fracture in Physically Active Young Servicemembers, December 10, Washington, D.C.

Shaffer, R.A., S.K. Brodine, and C. Corwin et al. 1994. Impact of musculoskeletal injury due to rigorous physical activity during U.S. Marine Corps basic training. Med. Sci. Sports Exerc. 26:S141.

Shane, E., M. Rivas, T.S. Kim, R.B. Staron, and D. Mancini. 1997. Bone loss and turnover after cardiac transplantation. J. Clin. Endocrinol. Metab. 82:1497–1506.

Shargil, A.A. 1985. Hormone replacement therapy in perimenopausal women with a triphasic contraceptive compound: A 3-year prospective study. Int. J. Fertil. 30:15–28.

Slemenda, C.W., S.L. Hui, C. Longcope, and CC Johnston Jr. 1989. Cigarette smoking, obesity, and bone mass. J. Bone Miner. Res. 4:737–741.

Slemenda, C.W., J.C. Christian, T. Reed, T.K. Reister, C.J. Williams, and C.C. Johnson Jr. 1992. Long-term bone loss in men: Effects of genetic and environmental factors. Ann. Intern. Med. 117:286–291.

Slootweg, M.C., D. Swolin, J.C. Netelenbos, O.G.P. Isaksson, and C. Ohlsson. 1997. Estrogen enhances growth hormone receptor expression and growth hormone action in rat osteosarcoma cells and human osteoblast-like cells. J. Endocrinol. 155:159–164.

Specker, B.L. 1996. Evidence for an interaction between calcium intake and physical activity on changes in bone mineral density. J. Bone Miner. Res. 11:1539–1544.

Stacy, R.J. and R.L. Hungeford. 1984. A method to reduce work-related injuries during basic recruit training in the New Zealand Army. Mil. Med. 149(6):318–320.

Stern, P.H. 1996. Thyroid hormone and bone. Pp. 521–531 in Principles of Bone Biology, J.P. Bilezikian, L.G. Raisz, and G.A. Rodan, eds. San Diego, Calif.: Academic Press, Inc.

Stevenson, J.C., M.P. Cust, and K.F. Gangar. 1990. Effects of transdermal versus oral hormone replacement therapy on bone density in spine and proximal femur in postmenopausal women. Lancet 335:265–269.

Stoneman, P. 1997. Rehabilitation of stress fractures in Army basic trainees. Presentation at the workshop on Reducing Stress Fracture in Physically Active Young Servicemembers, December 10, Washington, D.C.

Straus, F.H. 1932. Marching fractures of metatarsal bones with a report of the pathology. Surg. Gynec. Obstet. 54:581–584.

Sundgot-Borgen, T. 1993. Prevalence of eating disorders in elite female athletes. Int. J. Sports Nutr. 3:29–40.

Suominen, H. 1993. Bone mineral density and long-term exercise: An overview of cross-sectional athlete studies. Sports Med. 16:316–330.

Surrey, E.S., J.C. Gambone, and J.K.H. Lu. 1990. The effects of combining norethindrone with a gonadotropin-releasing hormone agonist in the treatment of symptomatic endometriosis. Fertil. Steril. 53:620–626.

Svendsen, O., C. Hassager, and C. Christiansen. 1993. Effects of an energy-restrictive diet, with or without exercise, on lean tissue mass, resting metabolic rate, cardiovascular risk factors, and bone in overweight postmenopausal women. Am. J. Med. 95:131–140.

Sweet, D.E., and R.M. Allman. 1971. RPC of the month from the AFIP. Radiology 99(3):687–693·

Taafe, D.R., T.L. Robinson, C.M. Snow, and R. Marcus. 1997. High-impact exercise promotes bone gain in well-trained female athletes. J. Bone Miner. Res. 12:255–260.

Teegarden, D., W.R. Prouls, B.R. Martin, J. Zhao, G.P. McCabe, R.M. Lyle, M. Peacock, C. Slemenda, C.C. Johnston, and C.M. Weaver. 1995. Peak bone mass in young women. J. Bone Miner. Res. 10:711–715.

U.S. Army Recruiting Command. 1998. Army Regulation 601-95. "Delayed Entry and Delayed Training Program." January 1. Fort Knox, Kentucky.

U.S. Department of Defense. 1995a. Department of Defense Directive 1308.1 "Physical Fitness and Body Fat Programs." July 20. Washington, D.C.

U.S. Department of Defense. 1995b. Department of Defense Instruction 1308.3. "Physical Fitness and Body Fat Programs Procedures." August 30. Washington, D.C.

U.S. Department of the Army. 1986. Army Regulation 600-9. "The Army Weight Control Program." September 1. Washington, D.C.

U.S. Departments of the Army, the Navy, and the Air Force. 1985. Army Regulation 40-25/Navy Command Medical Instruction 10110.1/Air Force Regulation 160-95. "Nutritional Allowances, Standards, and Education." May 15. Washington, D.C.

Volpe, A., M. Silferi, A.D. Genazzani, and A.R. Genazzani. 1993. Contraception in older woman. Contraception 47:229–239.

Wade, G.N., and J.E. Schneider. 1992. Metabolic fuels and reproduction in female mammals. Neurosci. Biobehav. Rev. 16:235–272.

Weaver, C. 1997. Calcium and Iron: Food vs. Supplements. Presentation at the workshop on Reducing Stress Fracture in Physically Active Young Servicemembers, December 10, Washington, D.C.

Westphal, K.A., K.E. Friedl, M.A. Sharp, N. King, T.R. Kramer, K.L. Reynolds, and L.J. Marchitelli. 1995. Health, performance, and nutritional status of U.S. Army women during basic combat training. Technical Report No. T96-2. Natick, Mass.: U.S. Army Research Institute of Environmental Medicine.

Williams, N.I., J.C. Young, J.W. McArthur, B. Bullen, G.S. Skrinar, and B. Turnbull. Strenuous exercise with caloric restriction: effect on luteinizing hormone secretion. Med. Sci. Sports Exerc. 27:1390–1398, 1995.

Wosk, J., and A. Voloshin. 1981. Wave attenuation in skeletons of young healthy persons. J. Biomech. 14(4):261–267.

Young, N., C. Formica, G. Szmukler, and E. Seeman. 1994. Bone density at weight-bearing and nonweight-bearing sites in ballet dancers: The effects of exercise, hypogonadism, and body weight. J. Clin. Endocrinol. Metab. 78:449–454.

Zernicke, R., J. McNitt-Gray, C. Otic et al. 1993. Stress fracture risk assessment among elite collegiate women runners. Pages 1506–1507 in Proceedings of the International Society of Biomechanics XIVth Congress, Paris.

A

Workshop Agenda and Abstracts

WORKSHOP AGENDA

REDUCING STRESS FRACTURE IN PHYSICALLY ACTIVE YOUNG SERVICEMEMBERS

A Symposium Sponsored by
Committee on Body Composition, Nutrition, and Health of Military Women
Food and Nutrition Board

December 10, 1997
National Academy of Sciences Auditorium
Washington, D.C.

AGENDA

8:30 A.M.–8:40 A.M.	Welcome on Behalf of the Committee on Body Composition, Nutrition, and Health of Military Women *Barbara O. Schneeman, Chair*

8:40 A.M.–8:50 A.M. Welcome on Behalf of the Food and Nutrition Board
Allison A. Yates, Director, Food and Nutrition Board

8:50 A.M.–9:00 A.M. Welcome on Behalf of the Military
LTC Karl E. Friedl, U.S. Army Medical Research and Materiel Command, Fort Detrick, Frederick, MD

I. Stress Fracture Incidence in Military Training

9:00 A.M.–9:30 A.M. Stress Fracture among Physically Active Women in the General Population
Peter Brukner, Stanford University, Stanford, CA

9:30 A.M.–9:50 A.M. Physical Training Interventions to Reduce Stress Fracture Incidence in Navy and Marine Corps Recruit Training
CDR Richard A. Shaffer, * *Naval Health Research Center, San Diego, CA*

9:50 A.M.–10:10 A.M. Rehabilitation of Stress Fractures in Army Basic Trainees
CPT Paul Durant Stoneman, Fitness Training Company, Fort Jackson, SC

10:10 A.M.–10:25 A.M. Part I Panel Discussion
Moderated by Anne Looker

10:25 A.M.–10:40 A.M. Break

II. Body Composition (weight, bone mineral content, muscle mass), Genetics, and Stress Fracture

10:40 A.M.–11:10 A.M. Procollagen Gene Mutations as a Predisposing Factor for Stress Fracture
Eitan Friedman, * *Chaim Sheba Medical Center, Tel-Hashomer, Israel*

11:10 A.M.–11:30 A.M. Structural Indices of Stress Fracture Susceptibility in Female Military Recruits
Thomas J. Beck, * *The Johns Hopkins University Outpatient Center, Baltimore, MD*

---

* Recipients of Defense Women's Health Research Program grants.

11:30 A.M.–11:50 A.M.	Quantitative Ultrasound and Other Risk Factors for Stress Fracture during Basic Training in Female U.S. Army Recruits *Donald B. Kimmel,* Merck Research Laboratories, West Point, PA*
11:50 A.M.–12:05 P.M.	Part II Panel Discussion *Moderated by Steven B. Heymsfield*
12:05 P.M.–1:00 P.M.	*Lunch* available in refectory

III. DIET AND PHYSICAL ACTIVITY

1:00 P.M.–1:30 P.M.	Calcium Intake and Exercise Level: Synergistic Effects on Bone *Bonny L. Specker, South Dakota State University, Brookings*
1:30 P.M.–2:00 P.M.	Calcium and Iron: Foods vs. Supplements *Connie M. Weaver, Purdue University, West Lafayette, IN*
2:00 P.M.–2:20 P.M.	Dietary Calcium and Related Nutrient Intakes in Military Men and Women *LTC John P. Warber, U.S. Army Research Institute of Environmental Medicine, Natick, MA*
2:20 P.M.–2:40 P.M.	Effects of Prolonged Inactivity on the Musculoskeletal System with Evaluation of Countermeasures *Steven R. Smith, Pennington Biomedical Research Center, Baton Rouge, LA*
2:40 P.M.–2:55 P.M.	Part III Panel Discussion *Moderated by Nancy F. Butte*
2:55 P.M.–3:05 P.M.	Break

IV. HORMONAL FUNCTION (AMENORRHEA, PREGNANCY) AND BONE HEALTH

3:05 P.M.–3:35 P.M.	Effect of Modulators of Bone Turnover on Changes in Markers of Bone Turnover *Michael Kleerekoper, Wayne State University, Detroit, MI*
3:35 P.M.–4:05 P.M.	IGF-1, Muscle Mass, and Bone Density *Clifford J. Rosen, St. Joseph Hospital and Maine Center for Osteoporosis Research and Education, Bangor*

4:05 P.M.–4:25 P.M.	Dietary Energy Requirements in Physically Active Men and Women: Threshold Effects on Reproductive Function *Anne B. Loucks,* Ohio University, Athens*
4:25 P.M.–4:45 P.M.	Fitness, Bone Density, and Injury and Illness in Postpartum Soldiers *COL Joseph R. Dettori,* Madigan Army Medical Center, Tacoma, WA*
4:45 P.M.–5:00 P.M.	Part IV Panel Discussion *Moderated by Gail E. Butterfield*
5:00 P.M.–5:30 P.M.	General Discussion *Moderated by Barbara O. Schneeman*
5:30 P.M.	Closing Remarks *Barbara O. Schneeman*

Reception for committee and military liaison panel members and speakers immediately following in the Rotunda

Dinner for committee and military liaison panel members and speakers following reception in the Members Room

Presentation: The Art and Science of Longitudinal Studies of Healthy Young People
Tom Lloyd, The Pennsylvania State University College of Medicine, Hershey Medical Center

WORKSHOP ABSTRACTS

The abstracts appear in the order in which they were presented during the workshop on "Reducing Stress Fracture in Physically Active Young Service Members" which was held on December 10, 1997, in Washington, D.C.

STRESS FRACTURE AMONG PHYSICALLY ACTIVE WOMEN IN THE GENERAL POPULATION

Peter Brukner, M.B., B.S., FACSP, FACSM, Stanford University, Stanford, CA 94306-6175 and Olympic Park Sports Medicine Centre, Melbourne, Australia

It is often suggested that women sustain a disproportionately higher number of stress fractures than men. Military studies consistently show that female recruits have a greater risk of stress fracture than to male recruits, with relative risks ranging from 1.2 to 10. This finding of an increased risk in women persisted even when training loads were applied gradually to a moderate level and when age and race were controlled. Possible reasons for a gender difference in stress fracture risk include differences in bone density, bone geometry, gait, biomechanical features, body composition, and endocrine factors, particularly estrogen status. In contrast, a gender difference in stress fracture rates is not as evident from athletic studies. These either show no difference between male and female athletes or a slightly increased risk for women, up to 3.5 times that of men. It is possible that a gender difference in stress fracture risk is lessened in athletes, as female athletes may be more conditioned to exercise than female recruits.

Twin studies have indicated that up to 90 percent of the variation in bone mass can be attributed to genetic factors. A significant relationship between a family history of osteoporosis and yearly change in bone density has been demonstrated in runners and nonrunners. Although it is feasible that some individuals may be genetically predisposed to stress fractures when exposed to suitable environmental conditions, such as vigorous exercise, there are few data to evaluate the role of genetic factors in predisposing an athlete to this injury.

Results of studies investigating the relationship between bone density and stress fracture risk have been contradictory. In a 12-mo prospective cohort study, female athletes who sustained tibial stress fractures had 8.1 percent less bone mass at the tibia/fibula. This finding was not evident for the male athletes. A large prospective study in the Israeli army and a cross-sectional study in athletes failed to corroborate a relationship between lower limb bone density and stress fractures.

Dietary factors, in particular calcium levels, may contribute to the development of stress fractures via influences on bone density and bone remodeling. In animal studies, a calcium-deficient diet decreased the ability of bone to adapt to mechanical strain, while high dietary calcium intake had a favorable effect on bone biomechanical properties. In humans, some studies have found a positive relationship between dietary calcium intake and bone mass, while others have noted small gains in bone mass resulting from calcium supplementation. There is conflicting evidence to show that low calcium intakes are associated with an increased risk for stress fracture in athletes. Other compounds such as protein, total energy, phosphorus, fiber, sodium, alcohol, and caffeine could potentially affect bone health and therefore stress fracture risk. At present, no associations have been found between these and the incidence of stress fractures in athletes. Dietary behaviors and eating patterns may differ in those with stress fractures. Studies have suggested that disordered patterns of eating may be associated with a higher risk for stress fracture. Whether this association is causal or due to some other factor is not clear.

Anthropometric characteristics, such as height and weight, and soft tissue composition, such as lean mass and fat mass, could theoretically affect stress fracture risk directly by influencing the forces applied to bones or indirectly via effects on bone density and menstrual function. No studies have compared muscle mass or muscle strength, particularly peak force production and fatigability, in athletes with and without stress fractures. No studies have reported differences in height, weight, body mass index, or fat mass among athletes who have and have not sustained a stress fracture.

PHYSICAL TRAINING INTERVENTIONS TO REDUCE STRESS FRACTURE INCIDENCE IN NAVY AND MARINE CORPS RECRUIT TRAINING

CDR Richard A. Shaffer, MSC, USN, Ph.D., M.P.H., Naval Health Research Center, San Diego, CA 92186

Introduction

Stress fractures during military training have a high fiscal and operational impact in Navy and Marine Corps populations. The incidence of reported stress fractures in males ranges from 0.2 percent in Navy recruits to 4.5 percent in Marine Corps recruits. The reported female incidence ranges from 0.7 percent in Navy recruits to 9.6 percent in Marine officer candidates. The estimated annual impact among 2,000 female Marine recruits is $1,850,000, with 4,120 lost training days.

Ongoing Research

Two studies are currently under way among female Marine Corps recruits to predict and prevent stress fractures during training. The goal of the first study is to develop and evaluate modifications to the physical training curriculum to reduce stress fractures. The second study is a collaborative Defense Women's Health Research Project (DWHRP) effort with The Johns Hopkins University to develop structural indices of stress fracture susceptibility. Both of these studies were follow-on studies to an initial DWHRP effort to determine risk factors for stress fracture among female recruits.

Conclusions

- Reported stress fractures have a higher impact on female training programs than on male programs.
- A significant factor affecting the increased rate of documented stress fractures in military women is differences in symptom reporting.
- Approximately 50 percent of stress fractures in military women are located on the femur and pelvis. These fractures result in greater rehabilitation time, disability, and operational costs compared to stress fractures below the knee.

• Stress fractures among women during military training are strongly associated with decreased levels of pretraining fitness and amounts of physical activity. Other specific risk factors are currently under investigation in these populations.

• In male military recruit populations, stress fractures have been reduced by 50 percent, without a decrease in graduation fitness, through the implementation of a safe and effective physical training curriculum. This curriculum was based on the fitness and activity attributes of the incoming recruit population.

• In female Navy recruits, a similar curriculum was designed that resulted in a 49 percent decrease in lower extremity overuse injuries.

• Physical training modifications, based on identified risk factors and military training goals, are under development for female Marine Corps recruits.

STRESS FRACTURE EXPERIENCE AT FORT JACKSON

CPT Paul Stoneman, M.S., USA, Fitness Training Company, 120th Adjutant General Battalion, Fort Jackson, SC 29207

Introduction

Fort Jackson is the largest integrated Army basic combat training (BCT) site. Over 40,000 soldiers were trained at Fort Jackson in FY1997. The physical demands of BCT can result in injury. The stress fracture is of particular concern because that type of injury has prolonged healing time, severely restricts the training ability of the injured soldier, and creates a host of administrative problems for the command.

Physical Training and Rehabilitation Program

In 1995, a Physical Training and Rehabilitation Program (PTRP) was created at Fort Jackson to help deal with the problem of soldiers injured in BCT who require extended recovery and rehabilitation. The majority of these soldiers have stress fractures of the lower extremities. Injured soldiers are pulled from the training unit and reassigned to PTRP for rehabilitation until they either return and complete BCT or are separated from the Army.

Experience and Interesting Observations

Our experiences at PTRP agree with the general findings of studies of injury patterns in military trainees:

- Stress fractures require prolonged recovery, often 60 days or more.
- Women are more at risk for injury, including stress fractures.
- Women are slightly less likely to recover and graduate from BCT once injured.

Interventions

Recently at Fort Jackson, a task force was formed to investigate injury prevention and management. Another group looked at the remedial physical training policy. A database is being developed to help track injuries sustained in BCT. Other actions include a trial of placing equipment, such as stationary cycles and strength-training equipment, in the training units. This equipment will be used by soldiers with specific needs, such as the less-fit soldier or the injured soldier. It has been shown that less-fit soldiers, either male or female, are more likely to be injured. Perhaps having such equipment in the training units will help the injured stay fit, return to training quicker, and provide resources for "cross-training" of the less-fit soldier.

IS THERE A GENETIC BASIS FOR STRESS FRACTURES?

Eitan Friedman, M.D., Ph.D.; Liat Ries, M.Sc.; Galia Yablonski-Gat, Ph.D.; Iris Vered, M.D.; Uri Givon, M.D.; and Joshua Shemer, M.D., The Suzanne Levy Oncogenetics Unit and the Endocrine Institute, Sheba Medical Center and the Medical Corps, IDF, Israel

Several lines of indirect evidence made it plausible (and testable) that in a subset of soldiers with stress fractures, there may be a genetic component. We initially hypothesized that subtle mutations in one of the two genes coding for procollagen type 1 genes that underly *Oseteogenesis imperfecta* may predispose to stress fractures. Under normal circumstances, these mutations would not result in any phenotype but manifest as stress fractures given the special workload placed on young, training soldiers. Several other genes may also be considered as candidate genes to be involved in the genetic predisposition to stress fractures, primarily those that are involved in pathological bone conditions and osteoporosis: vitamin D receptor, estrogen receptor, and calcium sensing receptor. This candidate gene approach was chosen for the lack of known multigenerational families with a definable pattern of stress fractures inheritance.

To test this hypothesis, IDF soldiers with clear evidence of high-grade stress fractures were identified. All pertinent data from these individuals (clinical, epidemiological, biochemical analysis of bone turnover parameters, and bone scan data) were obtained. In addition, constitutional DNA was extracted from peripheral blood leukocytes and analyzed for the existence of mutations within the above mentioned candidate genes by polymerase chain reaction (PCR) amplification, denaturing gradient gel electrophoresis (DGGE), DNA sequencing, and restriction enzyme digest of the relevant PCR products. As controls, two groups of soldiers were used: (1) a symptomatic control group composed of age-matched controls with no objective evidence of stress fractures, and (2) unit- and ethnicity-matched controls at the final stages of their basic training who were totally asymptomatic. The latter group completed the detailed questionnaire but underwent no bone scan or DNA testing. Results of the epidemiological and biochemical analyses will be presented in brief. Informed consent was given by 389 individuals, and blood was withdrawn from for DNA extraction. DNA was extracted from 200 soldiers. PCR amplification and DGGE analysis of 11 exons of the *COL1A1* (exons 3, 4, 6, 8, 11, 12, 13, 14, 15, 16, 50) and 7 of the *COL1A2* (exons 6, 10, 11, 12, 27, 29, 33) were done on all 200 samples. During these analyses, an abnormal migration pattern was detected in six samples in exon 12 of the *COL1A2* gene and found to be a base change that could lead to an alternative splicing. Moreover, a mutation within a glycine residue was detected in a single patient with osteogenesis imperfecta (OI). In addition, 160 soldiers underwent the vitamin D receptor analysis, and 80 soldiers underwent calcium-sensing receptor and an estrogen receptor novel polymorphism. The results of these genetic analyses, including statistical significance workup, were presented and discussed as a more comprehensive method of evaluating of the genetic component to stress fractures.

STRUCTURAL INDICES OF STRESS FRACTURE SUSCEPTIBILITY IN FEMALE MILITARY RECRUITS

T.J. Beck, C.B. Ruff, R.A. Shaffer, K. Betsinger, D.W. Trone, and S. Brodine*

Introduction

Intense military physical training subjects the bones of the lower limb to repetitive bending and torsional stresses that can lead to failure or stress fracture. Because not every military recruit suffers a stress fracture during training suggests that individuals with stress fractures have weaker bones. From an engineering standpoint, this means either that bones of fracture cases bend and twist more easily in training (i.e., producing greater mechanical stresses) or that their bones are made of a weaker material that fails more easily. Studies of Israeli Army (Milgrom et al., 1989) and male U.S. Marine Corps recruits (Beck et al., 1996) support the hypothesis that stress fracture susceptibility is due to geometric factors that determine mechanical stress magnitudes. In this study, dual energy x-ray absorptiometry (DXA) methods were used in male Marine Corps recruits (Beck et al., 1996) to determine whether the same bone geometric factors determine susceptibility in female Marine Corps recruits. Muscle strength may also be a factor in stress fracture susceptibility, since contraction of certain muscle groups tends to resist bending and twisting of long bones protectively. DXA scanners can also measure muscle mass; hence, the method was extended to determine if lower muscle mass was a contributing factor, since weaker muscles may compromise protection by fatiguing more easily.

Materials and Methods

A total of 671 female U.S. Marine Corps recruits at the Parris Island Recruit Depot were enrolled prior to onset of training. Using a Norland XR26 scanner (Norland Inc., Fort Atkinson, Wis.), DXA scans were obtained at the mid femur and distal third of the lower leg of the right side. A series of anthropometric measurements was also obtained that included height; weight; body mass index; lengths of the thigh and tibia; and girths of the neck, waist, hip, and thigh, as well as breadths of the pelvis, hips, and bicondylar dimensions at the knee. Using programs described previously (Beck et al., 1996), DXA data were used to derive cross-sectional areas (CSA), moments of inertia (CSMI), and section moduli (Z) at scan locations in the femur, tibia, and fibula. In addition, the whole bone strength index (Selker and Carter, 1989) was calculated for each bone as the ratio of Z to bone length. Also, since critical failure may be related to cortical thickness, an estimate of mean cortical thickness

* The Johns Hopkins University Outpatient Center, Baltimore, MD 21287-0849

was computed. The soft tissue of the thigh within the femur scan region was employed to obtain a measurement of relative lean muscle mass using standard Norland software. Recruits were followed through the 12-wk training to ascertain stress fractures using standard diagnostic criteria.

Results

A total of 36 recruits (5.2 %) suffered stress fractures: 13 in the foot, 10 each in the pelvic girdle and lower leg, and 9 in the femur. Of the main three ethnic groups, equivalent stress fracture rates were observed among Whites and Hispanics (≈6.5 %), while the rate among Blacks was only 2.6 percent. Cases were pooled and measurements compared with nonfracture cases using a t-test. No anthropometric variable was significantly different between groups ($p > .05$). Conventional BMD and estimated cortical thickness were significantly smaller for fracture cases in the femur, tibia, and fibula. Cross-sectional geometry variables measured at the midshaft of the femur and distal third of the tibia were, except for tibial width, significantly smaller in cases than controls (see Table A-1). Interestingly, the cross-sectional properties of the nonweight-bearing fibula were not significantly different from controls (not shown). The DXA-measured fraction of lean muscle mass at the thigh also was significantly smaller in fracture cases, which suggests that subjects with fractures had less muscular thighs, although thigh girths were not significantly smaller.

TABLE A-1 Average Values for Femur and Tibia Stress Fracture Cases and Controls and Differences between Groups

	Femur			Tibia		
Parameter	Cases	Controls	% Diff.	Cases	Controls	% Diff.
BMD (g/cm^2)	1.296	1.371	–5.5	0.952	1.020	–6.7
CSA (cm^2)	2.630	2.860	–8.0	1.669	1.822	–8.4
CSMI (cm^4)	0.994	1.138	–12.7	0.472	0.532	–11.3
Width (cm)	2.140	2.200	–2.7	0.185	0.189	–2.1*
Section modulus (Z) (cm^3)	0.921	1.023	–10.0	0.502	0.556	–9.7
Strength index (Z/bone length)	1.829	2.012	–9.1	1.384	1.493	–7.3
Average cortical thickness (cm)	0.518	0.559	–7.3	0.359	0.392	–8.4
Thigh lean mass fraction	0.736	0.764	–3.7			

NOTE: BMD, bone mineral density; CSA, cross-sectional area; CSMI, moment of inertia; Z, section modulus.

* All differences are significant ($p < 0.05$) with the exception of tibia width.

Discussion and Conclusions

Unlike male stress fracture subjects, who were generally smaller in weight and stature (Beck et al., 1996), female fracture subjects were not significantly different in body size. Like males, however, the measured bones of the lower limbs tended to have lower bone mass density (BMD). The mechanical relevance of the lower BMD is evident in the smaller cross-sectional properties of the limb bones of individuals with fractures. Particularly relevant is the smaller bone strength index in female fracture cases, an observation also seen in male Marine Corps recruits. The strength index is based on the observation that the resistance of a bone to bending and twisting is directly dependent on the section modulus and inversely related to bone length (Selker and Carter, 1989) (i.e., long, skinny bones are weaker than short, wide ones). The fact that relative muscle mass in the thigh is significantly reduced in fracture cases supports the hypothesis that muscle strength is, at least in females, a factor in stress fracture susceptibility.

These geometric differences support the hypothesis that the bones of test subjects are weaker than controls because they undergo greater stress magnitudes during training. Moreover, the lower relative thigh muscle mass suggests a diminished capability of muscle to resist stresses during training. The anthropometric and DXA methodologies used in this study were designed to measure factors influencing mechanical stress but not material properties. These results, therefore, do not rule out a role for degraded material strength, possibly due to dietary or genetic deficiencies. For example, reduced BMD values may also result from decreased mineralization, which would degrade the material properties, but this cannot easily be determined by current methodologies.

A number of additional questions remain. What component of the geometric differences is genetic and what component is environmental? It is known that stress fracture is relatively infrequent in African Americans (Jones et al., 1989); indeed, in the current study, the stress fracture rate in African Americans was less than half of that in Hispanics or Whites. Further work is necessary to answer these questions. Examination of such environmental factors as prior physical activity is also worth study. Certainly, physical activity influences muscle mass and is also believed to improve the geometry of bones in ways that minimize stress (Cowin, 1989). The implication for younger populations is that bone can be strengthened by rigorous training. Unfortunately, information regarding the rates and magnitudes of such change and the factors influencing such change in humans are scanty. Whether pretraining exercise regimens can be designed to precondition bones to minimize stress fractures has yet to be determined.

References

Beck, T., C. Ruff, F. Mourtada, R. Shaffer, K. Maxwell-Williams, G. Kao, D. Sartoris, and S. Brodine. 1996. DXA derived structural geometry for stress fracture prediction in male U.S. Marine Corps recruits. J. Bone Miner. Res. 11:645–653.

Cowin, S., ed. 1989. The mechanical properties of cortical bone tissue. Pp. 97–127 in Bone Mechanics. Boca Raton, Fla.: CRC Press.

Jones, B.H., J.M. Harris, T.N. Vinh, and C. Rubin. 1989. Exercise-induced stress fractures and stress reactions of bone: Epidemiology, etiology, and classification. Exerc. Sport Sci. Rev. 17:379–422.

Milgrom, C., M. Giladi, A. Simkin, N. Rand, R. Kedem, H. Kashtan, M. Stein, and M. Gomori. 1989. The area moment of inertia of the tibia: A risk factor for stress fractures. J. Biomech. 22:1243–1248.

Selker, F., and D.R. Carter. 1989. Scaling of long bone fracture strength with animal mass. J. Biomech. 22:1175–1183.

QUANTITATIVE ULTRASOUND AND OTHER RISK FACTORS FOR STRESS FRACTURE DURING BASIC TRAINING IN FEMALE U.S. ARMY RECRUITS

D.B. Kimmel, * M.R. Stegman, M. White, M.J. Lauren, and L. Hise*

This presentation provides new information that can reduce stress fracture incidence in both soldiers and athletes. First, a new perspective will be provided that views stress fracture, like osteoporotic fracture, as an example of fragility fracture (Table A-2). Second, prospective and nested case-control study designs will provide new data from basic training recruits. Interpretation of the data will relate to recommendations for practical interventions.

Approximately 4,200 female Army recruits enrolled at Fort Leonard Wood, Missouri, between 8/25/95 and 7/15/96. They filled out a risk factors questionnaire (family history, height, and weight; past smoking [yes/no]; initial fitness [Physical Training score]; menstrual onset and regularity; birth control pills; current and lifetime calcium intake and general nutrition; corticosteroid usage). They were also measured by quantitative ultrasound of the calcaneus (QUS). Smoking history of at least half a pack daily for 3 months or the equivalent was considered positive. Subjects were then followed through 8 weeks of basic training for diagnoses of stress fracture and overuse injury requiring visit(s) to the Troop Medical Clinic. At the time of initial visit for stress fracture diagnosis, a second QUS measurement was obtained. Time-matched nonfracturing controls were also measured in a nested case-control study.

TABLE A-2 Parallels of Stress Fracture and Osteoporotic Fracture

Characteristic	Stress Fracture	Osteoporotic Fracture
Prevalence among genders	6:1 women	5:1 women
Specific groups	Soldiers/athletes	Older women
Minority occurrence	~5–10% in BT	~25–30% cumulative
Site specificity	Foot, leg, thigh	Spine, hip, wrist
Measurable risk	QUS	BMD, QUS
Fitness related	Aerobic/muscular fitness	Grip strength, falls
Trauma related	Activities of daily soldiering	activities of daily living
Individuals identifiable prospectively	No	No
Preventable/treatable	Yes	Yes
Animal models	No	Yes

NOTE: BT, basic training; QUS, quantitative ultrasound of the calcaneus; BMD, bone mineral density.

* *Department of Bone Biology/Osteoporosis, Merck Research Laboratories, West Point, PA 19486*

Prospective data were first analyzed by logistic regression with stress fracture as the dependent variable and QUS variables (BUA [broadband ultrasound attenuation], SOS [speed of sound]) or other risk factors as independent variables. Then the QUS relative risk (per standard deviation decrease) and confidence intervals were calculated. Means and relative risks are presented in Table A-3. For a subset of 840 soldiers, the risk factors were combined in one backwards logistic regression analysis. For the nested case-control study, change in QUS values as a function of time post-initial measurement were compared for stress fracture and control individuals using the Mann-Whitney test. Initial QUS values for groups of individuals suffering fractures of foot bones, tibia, and femur/pelvis, respectively, were also compared.

TABLE A-3 Means and Relative Risks (Independent) for Stress Fracture

Variable	PT Score	SOS (m/sec)	SMK
Mean ± SD	102 ± 57.6	1,514 ± 8.8	29%
RR	2.89*	2.33*	2.87*
(95% CI)	1.83–4.55	1.58–3.43	1.51–5.45

NOTE: PT, physical test; SOS, speed of sound; SMK, smoker; SD, standard deviation; RR, relative risk; CI, confidence interval

* Per standard deviation decrease.

The darkened bars in Figure A-1 are the values and confidence intervals when the factors are combined in the backwards logistic regression model; the light bars are for independent consideration. Although both BUA and SOS were measured, SOS proved to be a stronger predictor of stress fracture risk, leaving no significant contribution for BUA. Taken independently, only these three factors were significant for stress fracture. No other measured or lifestyle factor played a role. More importantly, there is little overlap among them when these three factors are considered in the same model.

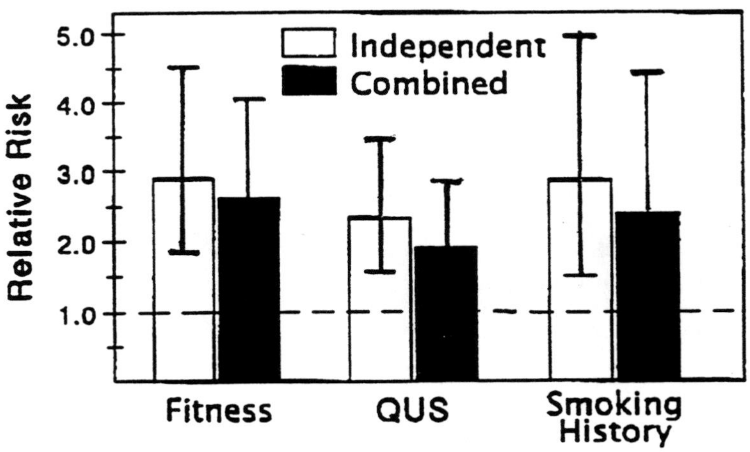

FIGURE A-1 Major risk factors for stress fracture in female U.S. Army soldiers.

A total of 332 soldiers with stress fractures and 448 control soldiers were evaluated in the nested case-control study by initial BUA and BUA at the time of visit 1 for stress fracture care. During the first 45 days of basic training, BUA declined more in stress fracture soldiers than in control soldiers (all $p < 0.005$) (Figure A-2). However, in soldiers measured during and after day 46 of training, BUA declined in neither group.

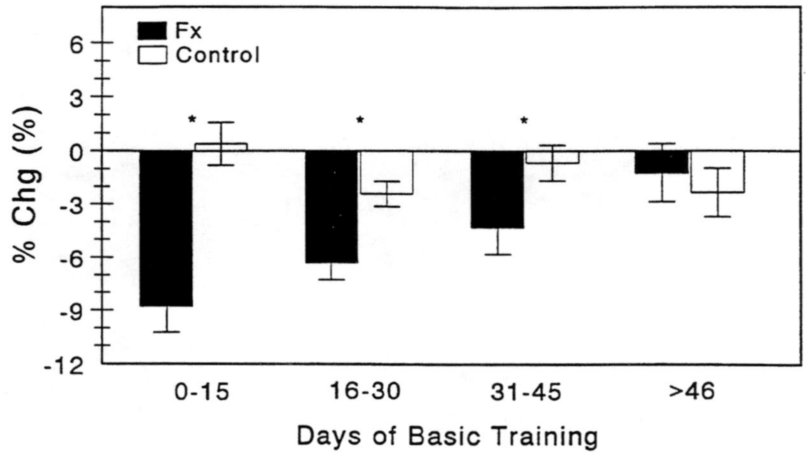

FIGURE A-2 Percentage change in broadband ultrasound attenuation from initial level.

Initial BUA in all three stress fracture groups was lower than in controls (all $p < 0.005$) (Figure A-3). However, initial BUA of soldiers with femoral or pelvis stress fracture was higher than that in soldiers with foot or tibial stress fracture ($p < 0.02$).

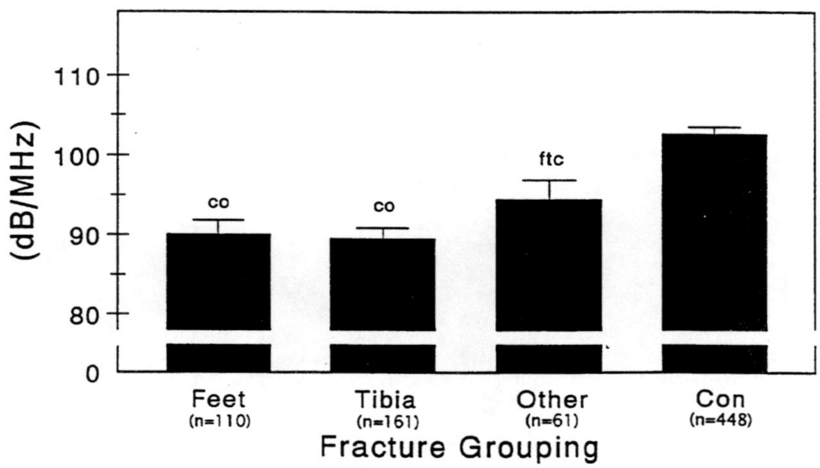

FIGURE A-3 Initial broadband ultrasound attenuation.

Both stress fracture during military basic training and osteoporotic fracture are examples of fragility fracture. Evaluating fitness, QUS, and smoking history—three independent determinants of stress fracture risk—gives a complete yet conveniently obtained picture of stress fracture risk in young, female soldiers. Although many other traditional risk factors for bone weakness were considered, it is likely that their influence is expressed by the QUS measurement. It remains impossible to predict perfectly stress fracture occurrence in individuals.

In conclusion, QUS measurement does not facilitate identification of individuals with a high risk of "high consequence" (e.g., proximal femur, pelvis) stress fracture. Moreover, QUS declines in stress fracture soldiers during basic training, indicating that those soldiers may respond to the increased physical activity of basic training with increased bone turnover that causes transient downward adjustment in bone strength due to an expansion of the remodeling space. This downward adjustment of bone strength may itself contribute to fracture occurrence.

CALCIUM INTAKE AND EXERCISE LEVEL: SYNERGISTIC EFFECTS ON BONE

Bonny L. Specker, Ph.D., South Dakota State University, Brookings, SD 57007

Both calcium intake and physical activity are thought to affect bone mass accretion early in life and bone loss later in life. However, results from randomized trials are not consistent. Results from a recently completed trial of gross motor activity during growth indicated that the effect of increased activity on bone mass accretion may be dependent on calcium intake. That is, decreased bone mass accretion was observed in individuals with a low calcium intake who were randomized to gross motor activities compared with those randomized to fine motor activities. In addition, 36 trials evaluating the effects of physical activity on changes in bone density in adults were reviewed. Studies were excluded if they did not include estimates of calcium intake. The studies were conducted in obese individuals; participants were noted to have significant changes in body weight, and/or bone sites not including the spine or radius were measured. A composite of the 16 studies meeting these criteria indicates that calcium intake and physical activity may not act on bone independently of each other. A beneficial effect of physical activity on bone appears to exist only at calcium intake greater than 1,000 mg/d. These results may explain inconsistent findings on the beneficial effects of either calcium intake or physical activity on bone mass.

CALCIUM AND IRON: FOOD VERSUS SUPPLEMENTS

Connie M. Weaver, PhD, Department of Foods and Nutrition, Purdue University, West Lafayette, IN 47907-1264

Mineral Requirements

Two nutrients that are most likely to be consumed at inadequate levels by the female military population are calcium and iron. The new calcium requirement for women aged 19 to 50 years, released in August 1997 by the Institute of Medicine is 1,000 mg/d. This recommended intake level is slightly above the ninetieth percentile of calcium intake based on the 1994 CFSII data. Thus, the majority of women are not consuming the recommended levels of calcium intake for optimal bone health. Peak bone mass in the hip is achieved by age 16 years and for the total body by the early 20s. Thus, adequate calcium protects against early bone loss rather than increasing peak bone mass after this age except for the spine, which can increase bone mass until age 30. A loss of 1 percent bone results in an increased risk of fracture of approximately 8 percent.

The Recommended Dietary Allowance for iron in menstruating women is 15 mg/d. This level of iron is difficult to achieve for most women, especially for those who restrict their intake of lean red meat.

Other minerals that may be inadequate in the female military population include magnesium and zinc. Evidence is mounting that adequate intakes of these nutrients are necessary for good bone health.

Bioavailability

Almost 75 percent of calcium in the American diet comes from dairy products. Other foods have much lower natural levels of calcium. Many plants also contain inhibitors to calcium absorption, notably oxalate and phytate. It would be extremely difficult to consume adequate calcium without consuming liberal quantities of dairy products, fortified foods, or supplements. Bioavailability of most calcium salts is equivalent to milk calcium.

Iron content and bioavailability are much greater in animal foods than in plant foods. Iron salts used to fortify foods vary widely in their bioavailability.

Nutrient-Nutrient Interactions

High sodium intakes and, to a lesser extent, high protein intakes increase urinary calcium losses. Some concern has been raised that high calcium intakes compromise iron, magnesium, and zinc status. Several recent studies have shown no harmful effects on magnesium status of up to 2 g/d of calcium intake. The harmful effects of calcium on iron status are shown in single-meal absorption studies. Chronic high calcium consumption has not been shown to compromise iron status, presumably because of upregulation of iron absorption. Reduced zinc retention has been documented at high calcium intakes in the elderly.

Foods Versus Supplements

Food patterns of fortification with milk extract have shown greater positive effects on bone than single nutrient interventions. Dairy foods provide a package of nutrients important for bone health. In the American diet, dairy products contribute 75 percent of the calcium, 35 percent of the riboflavin, 34 percent of the potassium, 20 percent of the magnesium, and 17 percent of the vitamin A, as well as being fortified with vitamin D. Because of this contribution and American's poor compliance with supplement regimens, supplements are not the first recommendation. However, supplementation may be indicated for individuals who do not otherwise meet their needs. Fortification with a package of nutrients may be a viable approach.

DIETARY CALCIUM AND RELATED NUTRIENT INTAKES IN MILITARY MEN AND WOMEN

LTC John P. Warber, USA, PhD, Nutrition and Biochemistry Division, U.S. Army Research Institute of Environmental Medicine, Natick, MA 01760-5007

Adequacy of nutrient intake by military personnel has been evaluated on a periodic basis since World War II. As new rations have been developed, their acceptability and relationship to performance have been studied. Few military nutrition monitoring studies have been conducted to determine how well military feeding addresses the nutritional requirements of military women. Approximately 14 percent of the active-duty Army population is women. Any investigations on military feeding and women have been done with Army personnel. Low intakes of calcium have been associated with higher risks for osteoporosis, hypertension, and colon cancer. The *Healthy People 2000* objective 2.8 calls for 50 percent of female youths less than 24 years of age to consume three or more servings of calcium-rich foods daily (about 900 mg calcium). The calcium standard established for military personnel subsisting under normal operating conditions (AR 40-25, 1985) is 800–1,200 mg. The higher value reflects the greater requirement for 17–18 year olds. The nutritional standard for operational rations (e.g., Meal, Ready-to-Eat; Tray Pack Rations) is 800 mg. The newly released Dietary Reference Intakes for calcium (1997) increase the recommended calcium intake to 1,000 mg/d.

Data on food consumption from six military dietary assessment studies between 1980 and 1995 showed female soldiers to have an average calcium intake of 924 mg. The average calcium intake reported by NHANES III and CSFII 1988–1991 for females of like age in the general population is 722 mg. The average calcium intake for males covering eight studies between 1987 and 1996 was 1,428 mg. The mean daily intake of calcium for males exceeded the Military Recommended Dietary Allowances (MRDA) in all dietary studies performed over the past 10 years. Mean daily intakes of phosphorus exceeded the upper level of the MRDA for females across all garrison studies and exceeded general population estimates for similar age categories (1,393 mg vs. 1,092 mg). The intake of phosphorus for males averaged 2,038 mg. The calcium to phosphorus ratios averaged 1:1.5 for females and 1:1.4 for males.

Based on data collected from a representative sample of over 3,000 soldiers who participated in the Army Food and Nutrition Survey (1997), female soldiers (n = 467) reported consuming a mean of 2.3 items from the dairy food group per day while male soldiers (n = 2,384) consumed 2.6 items. In general, female soldiers are slightly more aware than the general population of the relationship of dietary calcium intake to health. Seventy-nine percent of female soldiers versus 67 percent of the U.S. female population (USDA, *Diet and Health Knowledge Survey*, 1988–1991) identified inadequate calcium intake with the potential health outcome of osteoporosis, even though 50 percent of female soldiers believed their diets were too low in calcium. This underscores the need for research about what causes people to change their dietary behavior.

References

AR 40-25, 1985.

Army Food and Nutrition Survey, 1997.

Institute of Medicine (IOM). 1997. Dietary Reference Intakes.
Healthy People 2000.
USDA, Diet and Health Knowledge Survey, 1988-91.

EFFECTS OF PROLONGED INACTIVITY ON THE MUSCULOSKELETAL SYSTEM WITH EVALUATION OF COUNTERMEASURES

Steven R. Smith, M.D., Pennington Biomedical Research Center, Baton Rouge, LA 70808

Introduction

Prolonged inactivity is a component of many military missions and civilian occupations or circumstances. It is well recognized that these situations result in increased bone turnover, bone loss, nitrogen loss, and skeletal muscle deconditioning. A series of studies were conducted in vivo that focused on improving an existing catabolic model of inactivity and testing countermeasures to prevent nitrogen, muscle, and bone loss within the enhanced catabolic model.

Review

Prolonged bedrest, with the head lower than the feet, is an accepted model of spaceflight. These studies require 4 to 8 weeks to reach maximal calcium loss and typically are 17 weeks in duration. An improved model of bedrest catabolism was developed by combining 4 weeks of bedrest with low doses of thyroid hormone (triiodothyronine, T3). The model was compared with bedrest without T3 and shown to be superior to 4 weeks of bedrest alone. Specifically, bone turnover was increased, and calcium balance was more negative, with T3 treatment. Additional data on dynamic changes in markers of bone turnover complement calcium balance data and show that increases in bone resorption are a critical component of both bedrest and mild hyperthyroidism. Increases in bone formation occur late and are blunted relative to the increase in bone resorption. These studies then prompted a shift in focus to testing several countermeasures to prevent muscle and bone loss in the enhanced model. First, alendronate, a bisphosphonate inhibitor of bone resorption, was used concurrent with bedrest to prevent the increase in bone turnover and calciuria seen in the placebo-treated individuals. Testosterone was used as an anabolic agent to attenuate total-body nitrogen loss and losses of lean mass as measured by dual energy x-ray absorptiometry (DXA). Muscle strength was not preserved, however. Studies have recently been completed in 12 men to test a novel nutritional supplement, beta-hydroxy beta-methyl butyrate (HMB) to prevent loss of skeletal muscle. Previous studies have demonstrated a decrease in exercise-induced skeletal muscle turnover in healthy individuals treated with HMB, which suggests utility in states of increased protein flux.

Conclusions

Prolonged inactivity results in bone and muscle loss. Increased bone resorption is the primary mechanism by which calciuria occurs. The molecular mechanism(s) that increases bone resorption is unknown. Similarly, skeletal muscle protein turnover is increased via an unknown mechanism. These results demonstrate that skeletal muscle should be studied in a functional context, as preservation of mass does not necessarily preserve strength. The studies provide information useful for situations such as military missions requiring prolonged inactivity, postsurgical and/or postinjury immobility, inactivity associated with aging, and microgravity/spaceflight.

EFFECT OF MODULATORS OF BONE TURNOVER ON CHANGES IN MARKERS OF BONE TURNOVER

Michael Kleerekoper, M.D., Ph.D., Endocrine Division, Wayne State University, Detroit, MI 48201

Bone is subject to continuous turnover throughout life. This consists of removal of older bone (*resorption*) and replacement with new bone at the same site (*formation*). During growth and development, turnover is high, particularly in the first 2 years of life and again during the pubertal growth spurt. In these periods, formation exceeds resorption with accretion of bone and positive skeletal balance. Turnover, also termed *remodeling*, reaches a nadir as peak bone mass is attained during the third and fourth decades and the skeleton is in zero balance. After age 40, for unknown reasons, remodeling remains low, but resorption exceeds formation, and there is negative skeletal balance. With the menopause, there is an acceleration of remodeling with a greater excess of resorption over formation and more rapid negative balance. Turnover appears to slow down about 10 years postmenopause, only to accelerate again during the eighth decade and beyond. There are several markers of the resorption process, all of which are based on breakdown products of the bone matrix (type 1 collagen). These include the major amino acid hydroxyproline and the pyridinium cross-links of collagen. There are several markers of these cross-links: pyridinoline and deoxypyridinoline, and the amino- and carboxy-terminal telopeptides of these cross-links. Markers of bone formation are gene products of the osteoblast, bone-specific alkaline phosphatase, osteocalcin, and procollagen extension peptides. Many medical conditions and therapies modulate turnover, and these effects can be monitored by changes in the above markers. Generally, these reflect systemic events, including estrogen deficiency from any cause, thyroid, parathyroid, and cortisol excess from endogenous and exogenous sources; malnutrition and malabsorption; and immobilization. In military-age women, there is cause for concern about hypothalamic amenorrhea (excess exercise, anorexia, bulimia), and therapy with gonadotrophin-releasing hormone (GnRH) agonists that may be used in endometriosis. Contraceptives (oral and depot) may have adverse effects on the skeleton, but this is not yet firmly established, and the potential mechanisms are unclear. Local events such as traumatic, fragility, and stress fractures increase remodeling locally, but the assays may not be sensitive enough to detect this in all cases. It has been postulated that remodeling may be initiated at some sites as a means of repairing microdamage. If microdamage accumulates at a rate faster than can be corrected by remodeling processes, the damage propagates to demonstrable fracture. This may be the case with stress fractures, although it remains speculative. High rates of remodeling, as are seen during puberty, do not appear to result in stress fractures, so it is unlikely that systemically induced increases in remodeling will result in stress fractures. In contrast, local abnormalities in remodeling, particularly when formation is markedly increased, may be associated with local stress fractures. Examples include osteomalacia, Paget's disease of bone, and therapy with sodium fluoride. Because fluoride therapy only results in lower-extremity stress fractures, an apparent link exists between local factors predisposing to stress fractures and mechanical load bearing. The relevance of this link to stress fractures in the military remains speculative.

IGF-1, MUSCLE MASS, AND BONE DENSITY*

C.J. Rosen, W G. Beamer, L.R. Donahue, D.J. Baylink, J. Rogers, C.H. Turner, and J.P. Bilezikian, St. Joseph Hospital and Maine Center for Osteoporosis Research and Education, Bangor, ME 04401 and The Jackson Laboratory, J. L. Pettis VA Hospital, Southwest Foundation for Biomedical Research, Indian University Medical Center, and Columbia University, New York, NY.

Insulin-like growth factor (IGF)-I, a ubiquitous polypeptide induced by growth hormone, has traditionally been considered a critical element for the linear growth of mammals. However, IGF-1 is abundant in the adult skeleton and plays a central role in remodeling as well as in acquisition of peak bone mass. Moreover, growth hormone and IGF-1 are major determinants of lean body mass. In the circulation as well as in muscle and bone, tissue-specific IGF regulatory elements (e.g., IGF binding proteins [BPs], IGF receptors, IGFBP proteases) control the bioavailability of this potent growth factor. However, discerning the true functional relationship between IGF-1 and peak bone mass has been difficult for several reasons: (1) the lack of a good *in vivo* model, (2) the use of serum IGF-1 as a surrogate marker for tissue IGF-1, and (3) a host of confounding variables that affect IGF-1. Two model systems were used to examine the role of IGF-1 in musculoskeletal acquisition and maintenance: (1) males with the syndrome of idiopathic osteoporosis (IOM), and (2) healthy, inbred strains of mice. These authors recently described a cohort of men with osteoporosis who have low serum IGF-1 and reduced bone formation. In the syndrome of IOM, homozygosity in a simple sequence-length polymorphism (SSLP) of a nontranscribing region in the IGF-1 gene is considerably more frequent (65 %) than in a healthy control group (32 %) (O.R. 3.9, $p < 0.003$) and is associated with low serum IGF-1 levels in a random population of men, women, and pubertal girls. Coincident with these human studies, these authors recently reported large differences in both skeletal and serum IGF-1 in two inbred strains of mice. Using intercrosses to produce F2 progeny, it was noted that IGF-1 phenotype cosegregates with bone mass and accounts for 40 percent of the variance in bone mineral density (BMD). Currently, genes are being mapped that control serum IGF-1 through quantitative trait localization (QTL). Moreover, in functional experiments with a GH-deficient mouse (*little*), these authors have found that introducing a portion of the genome from a high-density, high IGF-1 mouse can markedly increase both BMD and serum IGF-1, despite the absence of growth hormone. These studies suggest that IGF-1 plays a major role in the acquisition and maintenance of bone mass. Through the use of congenic strains and QTLs for BMD, these laboratories are currently determining whether the genetic loci that regulate bone density are similar or identical to those that control tissue and serum IGF-1 expression. In addition to that genomic search, an examination has also begun of the difference in body composition between these two inbred strains. High IGF-1 (high-density) strains have greater muscle mass, uterine weights, and less fat than do the low IGF-1 (low-density) strain. Similarly, femur strength, toughness, failure load, and moment of inertia are markedly greater ($p <$

* Supported by grants from the U.S. Public Health Service and Department of Defense Health Research Program grants.

0.0001) in the high-density, high IGF-1 strain than in the low-density mice. These data suggest that IGF-1 may play a key role in determining peak bone mass, and the heritable differences in the expression of IGF-1 could determine musculoskeletal strength and balance. These findings, produced through the unique collaborative efforts of several investigators, may have future implications for screening recruits who are at high risk for subsequent stress fractures.

DIETARY ENERGY REQUIREMENTS IN PHYSICALLY ACTIVE MEN AND WOMEN: THRESHOLD EFFECTS ON REPRODUCTIVE FUNCTION

Anne B. Loucks, Ph.D., Department of Biological Sciences, Ohio University, Athens, OH 45701

The prevalence of amenorrhea is elevated in civilian and military women who restrict their diets and who are intensely physically active. The endocrine mechanism of this amenorrhea involves the disruption of luteinizing hormone (LH) pulsatility. This presentation shows preliminary results from a randomized, prospective experiment that is testing the following hypothesis:

1. LH pulsatility and energy metabolism are disrupted at an energy availability of 10 kcal/kg lean body mass (LBM)/d in women but not in men, and
2. LH pulsatility is disrupted abruptly at a particular threshold of energy availability in women.

In repeated trials, young, regularly menstruating, untrained women and young untrained men performed controlled exercise and consumed controlled diets differing in energy content for 5 days. The women were tested in the follicular phase of their menstrual cycles. In subjects who had energy availabilities of 45 and 10 kcal/kg LBM/d, low energy availability (defined as dietary energy intake minus exercise energy expenditure) appears to have (1) reduced plasma glucose while increasing serum β-hydroxybutyrate; (2) reduced serum T3, serum insulin-like growth factor (IGF)-I, and serum insulin while increasing serum cortisol, serum growth hormone (GH), and serum insulin-like growth factor binding protein (IGFBP)-1; (3) increased fat oxidation while reducing carbohydrate oxidation during rest and exercise; and (4) reduced 24-h LH pulse frequency while increasing LH pulse amplitude in women but not in men. These preliminary results suggest that low energy availability has similar metabolic effects in men and women as their bodies conserve glucose for the brain where LH pulsatility is controlled, but that women require more energy availability than men to maintain normal LH pulsatility, and therefore to maintain their reproductive and skeletal health.

EFFECT OF PREGNANCY ON THE FITNESS AND HEALTH OF POSTPARTUM SOLDIERS

COL Joseph R. Dettori, LTC (R) Kathleen Westphal, CPT Tony Pusateri, LTC (R) Alana Cline, COL (R) Paul Smith, Troy Patience, Rex Hoyt, Madigan Army Medical Center, Ft. Lewis, Tacoma, WA 98431-5000

Pregnant and postpartum soldiers have unique needs that require adjustments in the demands placed on them in a military environment. This prospective cohort study was undertaken to examine the effects of pregnancy on the fitness and health of postpartum soldiers. A total of 468 females were studied in three different groups: a nonpregnant, active-duty group (NPAD, $n = 215$); a postpartum, family member group (PPFM, $n = 126$); and a postpartum, active-duty group (PPAD, $n = 127$). Soldier fitness was assessed using scores from soldiers' semi-annual Army physical fitness test (APFT) immediately prior to study entry and 6 to 9 months later. Subjects underwent blood draws to assess calcium status, anthropometric measurements to determine body composition, and dual energy x-ray absorptiometry to measure bone mineral density (BMD) immediately postpartum and at 6 months follow-up. Medical records of active-duty subjects were reviewed between January 1, 1992, and study termination to calculate injury and illness rates at baseline (preconception) and during the various phases of postpartum recovery.

Results

Forty-eight percent of postpartum soldiers failed to return to their prepregnancy fitness level 6 to 9 months postpartum and were nearly four times more likely to fail their postpartum APFT compared with nonpregnant soldiers (relative risk (RR) = 3.89, 95% confidence interval (CI) = 1.61, 9.39). BMD decreased in the postpartum period by 2.1 percent and 1.9 percent in the lumbar spine and femoral neck, respectively, for nonnursing PPAD mothers ($p = 0.001$ and 0.0086, compared with NPAD) and 5.0 and 5.4 percent for nursing PPAD mothers ($p = < 0.0001$ and < 0.0001 compared with NPAD). For women not in basic combat training or advanced individual training, crude injury and illness rates were 7.3 and 18.0 per 100 soldiers per month, respectively. These rates increased in the postpartum period (RR = 1.37 for injury, 95% CI = 1.08, 1.75; RR = 1.24 for illness, 95% CI = 1.06, 1.46).

Conclusions

Postpartum soldiers in the year following delivery demonstrated significantly reduced fitness, increased injury and illness rates, and reduced trabecular BMD. More research is needed to determine the reasonableness of the U.S. Army's requirement to return postpartum soldiers to body fat standards and minimum military fitness 135 days postpartum. In addition, strategies that optimize the postpartum soldier's restoration to prepregnancy fitness should be explored.

THE ART AND SCIENCE OF LONGITUDINAL STUDIES OF HEALTHY YOUNG PEOPLE

Tom Lloyd, Ph.D., The Pennsylvania State University College of Medicine, Hershey Medical Center, Hershey, PA 17033

Osteoporosis prevention is currently at a delicate stage. Recognition that calcium intake by young American women declined markedly in the past three decades while the prevalence of osteoporosis among older women increased dramatically has led to widespread investigations of the relationships between calcium intake and bone health. However, current understanding of age-related calcium requirements and bone health—both of which are multifactorial—is inadequate at present.

Women gain approximately 50 percent of the bone mineral content of their skeleton during adolescence. However, adolescent women in the United States consume on average only 65 percent of the Recommended Dietary Allowance of 1,200 mg/d calcium. The advent of dual energy x-ray absorptiometry provided the key to designing a study to quantify bone changes in children and young women and to assess the effect of calcium supplementation.

The *Pennsylvania State Young Women's Health Study* is an ongoing National Institutes of Health-funded longitudinal study of cardiovascular, bone, and endocrine development in healthy, young women. The study was initiated in 1990 when the subjects were, on average, 12 years of age; they are now, on average, 19 years of age. A major initial objective of this study was to determine the effect of calcium supplementation on bone gain during adolescence.

During the 4 years of active intervention as the participants grew from age 12 to age 16, the calcium-supplemented group made significantly greater bone gains than did the placebo group. However, within 1 year after treatment, by age 17, the differences had largely disappeared as the placebo treated group "caught up." The definitive assessment of the effect of the calcium supplementation program on peak bone mass cannot be made until the study cohort has reached skeletal maturity. Because Caucasian women acquire at least 95 percent of their bone mass by age 20, the volunteers must be studied again at and after this age.

With regard to bone health, attention has been focused on fracture reduction, bone density has been used to reflect fracture risk. In fact, fractures occur when bone strength and bone microarchitecture diminish past some as yet poorly understood set of circumstances. Bone strength and architecture are much more than bone mass and bone density. Studies from sports and the workplace report that bone geometry and bone strength are affected by physical activity. bone geometry and the nonmineral bone components must now be studied for their roles in establishing bone strength.

Three important research design issues that are specific to longitudinal studies with healthy participants include: (1) the research design requires planning that often spans several years, (2) research teams are often large and multidisciplinary to take advantage of multiple measurements, and these teams must remain functional for many years, and (3) the success of longitudinal studies depends entirely on continuing retention of a large proportion of the study subjects. Longitudinal studies offer several advantages over cross-sectional investigations. These advantages include: (1) Measurement of the endpoint variables is generally better than with cross-sectional studies because the measurement technology is repeated, and often the same personnel are making the repeated measurements. (2) both intersubject and intrasubject variability can be estimated. Thus, longitudinal studies have greater statistical power to detect differences in group assignment or due to treatment effects. (3) Only longitudinal studies offer the opportunity to follow-up unexpected observations made during the collection of the primary outcome variables.

Strategies to retain healthy volunteers in longitudinal studies must be addressed in planning and conducting the study. For studies involving healthy young people, six strategic areas relate to participant retention: (1) incentives, (2) personal health knowledge and benefits, (3) social responsibility, (4) study ownership, (5) continuity of study personnel and continuity of study measurements, and (6) the use of noninvasive procedures. Careful attention to each of these areas has allowed this laboratory to retain 72 percent of the starting participants in the *Pennsylvania State Young Women's Health Study*.

B

Military Recommended Dietary Allowances (AR 40-25, 1985: Chapters 1 and 2)

Headquarters
Departments of the Army,
the Navy, and the Air Force
Washington, DC
15 May 1985

***Army Regulation 40-25/Naval Command Medical Instruction 10110.1/Air Force Regulation 160-95**

Medical Services

Nutrition Allowances, Standards, and Education

Summary. This joint regulation on nutrition allowances, standards, and education has been revised. It defines the nutrition responsibilities of The Surgeons General of the Army, the Navy, and the Air Force. This regulation—

a. Provides a current statement of the military recommended dietary allowances.

b. Sets nutrient standards for packaged rations.

c. Provides a standardized nutrient density index for normal and reduced calorie menu planning.

d. Provides nutrition education guidance to assist the military in promoting a healthful diet.

Applicability. This regulation applies to all active elements of the Army, Navy, and Air Force. It also applies to the Reserve Components of these Services.

Impact on New Manning System. This regulation does not contain information that affects the New Manning System.

Supplementation. Supplementation of and exceptions to this regulation are prohibited without prior approval from HQDA (DASG-PSP), WASH DC 20310-2300; Department of the Navy, Naval Medical Command, WASH DC 20732; or HQ USAF/SGB, Bolling AFB, WASH DC 20332-6188, for each respective Service. Nutrient standards prescribed in table 2-3 for operational and restricted rations are not subject to exception.

Interim changes. Interim changes to this regulation are not official unless they are authenticated by The Adjutant General, Headquarters, Department of the Army (HQDA). Users will destroy interim changes on their expiration dates unless sooner superseded or rescinded.

Suggested improvements. The Army office of primary interest in this regulation is the Office of The Surgeon General, HQDA. Army users are invited to send comments and suggested improvements on DA Form 2028 (Recommended Changes to Publications and Blank Forms) directly to HQDA (DASG-PSP),

WASH DC 20310-2300. Other users may send comments and recommendations through normal channels to their respective Surgeons General: Naval Medical Command, ATTN: MEDCOM-312, Navy Department, WASH DC 20372, for the NAVY; and HQ USAF/SGB, WASH DC 20332-6188, for the Air Force.

Contents

Chapter 1
Introduction

1-1. Purpose

This regulation defines the nutrition responsibilities of The Surgeons General of the Army, Navy, and Air Force by—

a. Establishing dietary allowances for military feeding.

b. Prescribing nutrient standards for packaged rations.

c. Providing, basic guidelines for nutrition education as prescribed in DOD 1338.10-M.

1-2. References

a. Required Publications.

(1) DOD Manual 1338.10-M, Manual for the Department of Defense Food Service Program. (Cited in para 1-1.)

(2) TB MED 507/NAVMED P-5052-5/AFP 160-1, Occupational and Environmental Health: Prevention, Treatment, and Control of Heat Injury. (Cited in para 2-5*i*.)

b. Related publications. (A related publication is merely a source of additional information. The user does not have to read it to understand this regulation.)

(1) *Recommended Dietary Allowances*, ninth revised edition, 1980. (Copies may be obtained from the Office of Publications, National Academy of Sciences, 2101 Constitution Avenue, WASH DC 20418.)

(2) United States Department of Agriculture Handbook 8 Series, *Composition of Foods, Raw, Processed, and Prepared.* (Copies may be obtained from the Superintendent of Documents, US Government Printing Office, WASH DC 20402.)

1-3. Explanation of abbreviations and terms

Abbreviations and special terms used in this regulation are explained in the glossary.

1-4. Responsibilities

a. The Surgeon General, Department of the Army (TSG, DA). TSG, DA, will act as the Department of Defense (DOD) Executive Agent for Nutrition and will—

(1) Establish dietary allowances for military personnel subsisting under normal operating conditions.

(2) Establish nutrient standards for packaged rations.

(3) Adjust dietary allowances and nutrient standards to meet variations in age, sex, body size, physical activity, climate, or other conditions that may influence nutritional requirements.

(4) Evaluate current and proposed operational rations. Recommend adjustments and other actions to ensure that the nutrient composition of the

rations as offered for consumption meets the nutritional requirements of personnel in all operational environments.

(5) Coordinate the development of nutrition education programs for all Services.

(6) Provide qualified representatives to advise committees which support the DOD Food Service Program in matters that affect the nutritional quality of the military diet.

b. The Surgeons General of the Army, Navy, and Air Force. TSGs will—

(1) Review requests and make appropriate recommendations for deviations from established nutritional standards.

(2) Evaluate adjustments to planned diets (menus). Make recommendations to ensure that the nutrient composition of the diet as offered will promote and maintain health.

(3) Evaluate the nutritional status of personnel and report nutritional deficiencies or excesses.

(4) Recommend standard methods to assess body composition.

(5) Provide nutritional guidance to the Services' weight control and physical fitness programs.

(6) Develop and implement a Service-wide nutrition education program for military personnel and their dependents. Provide information to motivate the consumption of a nutritionally adequate diet that contains all of the macronutrients and micronutrients needed to promote health and to maintain desirable body weight.

(7) Assist in providing food service personnel with knowledge and skills of proper food preparation that will maintain the nutritional value of foods.

(8) Provide qualified representatives to—

(a) Advise local food service organizations, such as menu boards, on matters that affect the nutritional quality of meals prepared and consumed.

(b) Serve as consultants to installation commanders on the development and evaluation of nutritional aspects of the Services' weight control and physical fitness programs.

Chapter 2
Nutritional Allowances and Standards

2-1. Military recommended dietary allowances

a. Table 2-1 prescribes military recommended dietary allowances (MRDA) for military personnel. These allowances are adapted from the National Academy of Sciences/National Research Council publication *Recommended*

Dietary Allowances (RDA), ninth revised edition, 1980. MRDA are the daily essential nutrient intake levels presently considered to meet the known nutritional needs of practically all 17- to 50-year old, moderately active military personnel.

b. MRDA are intended for use by professional personnel involved in menu planning, dietary evaluation on a population basis, nutrition education, nutrition research, and food research and development. MRDA are based on estimated nutritional requirements. They provide broad dietary guidelines for healthy military personnel.

c. MRDA represent recommended daily nutrient intake levels, which should meet the physiological requirements of nearly all healthy military personnel. The energy allowances shown in table 2-1 represent ranges of caloric intake reflecting wide variations in energy requirements among individuals at similar levels of activity. These energy allowances are designed to maintain desirable body weight for healthy service members under conditions of moderate physical activity in an environment compatible with thermal comfort. The allowances are not to be interpreted as individual requirements. Also, they may not apply to personnel requiring special dietary treatment for conditions such as infection, chronic disease, trauma, unusual stress, pregnancy, lactation, or weight reduction. The allowances are subject to adjustments as outlined in paragraphs 2-3 and 2-4.

d. MRDA refer to the nutrient concentrations of edible portions of food offered for consumption. Nutrient losses may occur during food processing and preparation. These nutrient losses must be considered when nutrient composition tables are used to compare menus or food products with these allowances. The most recent edition of the United States Department of Agriculture Handbook 8 series, *Composition of Foods, Raw, Processed, and Prepared,* will be used as the standard reference nutrient composition data base.

2-2. Estimated safe and adequate daily dietary intakes
Table 2-2 is based on the RDA and provides estimated safe and adequate adult dietary intake ranges for selected nutrients, which are known to be essential in the diet, but for which recommended levels of intake have not been established.

2-3. Nutrient standards for operational and restricted rations
Table 2-3 prescribes nutrient standards, which are the criteria for evaluating the nutritional adequacy of operational and restricted rations. Operational rations include the individual combat ration such as the meal, combat, individual (MCI); the meal, ready-to-eat (MRE); and other rations (A, B, or T) used to support operations in the field. A level of 3600 kilocalories (kcal) is required for operational rations to meet energy demands associated with extended field operations. (See para 2-4.) Total fat calories should not exceed 40 percent of

the energy value of the operational ration or 160 grams (gm). It is essential that ration planners compensate for losses of nutrients, such as ascorbic acid, thiamin, riboflavin, niacin, and pyridoxine (vitamin B6), which may occur during storage of operational and restricted rations.

a. Nutritionally complete, individual operational rations such as the MCI and MRE must be formulated so that the nutrient content of each day's ration satisfies these nutrient standards. It is desirable that each combat meal provides one-third of the nutrient standard.

b. Under certain operational scenarios such as long-range patrol, assault and reconnaissance, and other situations where resupply is unavailable, it may be necessary for troops to subsist for periods (up to 10 days) on a restricted ration. To minimize loss of performance, the restricted ration should provide 1100 to 1500 kilocalories, 50 to 70 grams of protein, and a minimum of 100 grams of carbohydrate on a daily basis. Vitamins and minerals should be provided at the levels prescribed in table 2-3. This restricted ration is not appropriate for use under extreme, cold climates.

c. The survival food packet is a packaged food bar of approximately 400 kilocalories derived from carbohydrates. The low protein content spares body water by reducing the obligatory water demand caused by consuming high protein foods. The nutrient standards for operational and restricted rations do not apply to the survival food packet. This packet is designed to be consumed for periods of less than 4 consecutive days.

2-4. Energy requirements

The following factors affect individual energy requirements:

a. Age. MRDA are intended for men and women 17 to 50 years of age. Upon completion of growth, energy requirements for adults gradually decline with age due to a reduced resting metabolic rate and curtailment in physical activity. Within the 17 to 50 year military age range, age-related differences in caloric allowances appear to be minimal under conditions of similar physical activity.

b. Body size. The energy allowances are established for average sized personnel, which represent approximately 70 percent of the military personnel between the ages of 17 and 50 years. (See table 2-1.) To maintain desirable body weight, caloric intake must be adjusted for variable energy requirements due to individual differences in lean body mass reflected by body size. Large individuals (such as those with greater height and appropriately higher weight) have slightly higher resting, basal metabolic rates. They, therefore, require more total energy per unit of time for activities that involve moving body mass over distance. Smaller sized individuals require fewer calories.

c. Physical activity. Differences in energy needs are largely due to differences in the amount of time an individual performs moderate and heavy work tasks in contrast to light or sedentary activities. MRDA for energy in table 2-1 are for military personnel who are moderately active and living in a temperate climate or in a thermally neutral environment. Total energy requirements are influenced by the intensity and duration of physical activity. For example, a day of moderate physical activity may include 8 hours of sleeping, 12 hours of light activity, and 4 hours of moderate to heavy activity. For military personnel doing heavy work or involved in prolonged, vigorous physical training, the recommended caloric allowance should be increased by at least 25 percent (approximately 500 to 900 kilocalories).

d. Climate. MRDA for energy intake are established for personnel in a temperate climate. (See table 2-1.) When there is prolonged exposure to cold or heat, energy allowances may need adjustment.

(1) *Cold environment.* In a cold environment (mean temperature less than 14 °C (57.2 °F), the energy cost of work for garrison troops is approximately 5 percent greater than in a warmer environment. There is an additional 2 to 5 percent increase in energy expenditure associated with carrying the extra weight of heavy, cold weather clothing and footgear (the "hobbling" effect). Garrison personnel may require an extra 150 to 350 kilocalories per day under these conditions. Energy allowances of 4500 calories for men and 3500 calories for women are required to support adequately clothed troops maneuvering for prolonged periods (several hours) with heavy gear on foot, snowshoes, and skis over snow- or ice-covered terrain. This increased energy allowance does not apply to troops stationed in cold climates who are engaged in moderate activity within a garrison setting.

(2) *Hot environment.* In a hot climate, loss of appetite may cause a voluntary but undesirable reduction in caloric intake below the level of need. This loss of appetite may be most noticeable after troops have arrived in a hot environment and before the process of acclimatization is completed. When personnel are required to perform the same amount of work in a hot environment as in a temperate environment, the caloric expenditure will be increased. Little adjustment appears to be necessary for a change in environmental temperature between 20 °C (68 °F) and 30 °C (86 °F). It is desirable under conditions of moderate physical activity to increase the caloric allowance by at least 0.7 percent for every degree centigrade rise in average ambient temperature above 30 °C (86 °F). Daily energy requirements under extremely hot conditions (greater than 40 °C (104 °F), may reach 56 kcal/kilogram (kg) of body weight.

(3) *Nuclear, biochemical, and chemical environment.* Certain conditions will require special guidance and nutrient formulation not described in this regulation. One such condition is when troops are operating in contaminated environments for more than 6 hours while wearing protective clothing.

2-5. Nutrient discussion

a. Protein. MRDA for protein are based, in part, on an estimated nutritional requirement of 0.8 gm/day/kg of body weight. (See table 2- 1.) For military personnel within the reference weight range, protein recommendations are set between 48 to 63 gm/ day, for males and 37 to 50 gm/day for females. These computed protein levels have been further increased to 100 gm/day for male and 80 gm/day for female personnel. This increase reflects usual intake patterns and helps to maintain a high level of palatability and food acceptance among military personnel. These allowances are based on the consumption of a diet containing mixed proteins of animal and vegetable origin. A total day's protein intake of more than 100 gm/day has not been shown to improve heavy physical performance.

b. Fat. Fats are important in the diet to furnish energy, provide essential fatty acids, transport fat soluble vitamins and aid in their absorption, increase palatability, and give meal satisfaction. It is becoming increasingly clear that excessive amounts to total fat may lead to an increased risk of coronary heart and vascular disease. For this reason, it is recommended that the calories derived from total dietary fat should not exceed 35 percent under garrison feeding conditions. Higher proportions of fat calories are acceptable in combat, arctic, or other operational rations to increase caloric density. Emphasis should be placed on planning the military menu with lower fat concentrations while maintaining acceptability. A reduction of fat calories in the diet can be achieved by lowering added fats during food preparation and replacing foods high in fat with lean meats, fish, poultry, low fat milk; and other low fat dairy products in the military menu. As fat calories are reduced in the diet, it is recommended that the current level of about 7 percent of caloric intake as polyunsaturated fat be maintained to ensure an adequate intake of essential fatty acids.

c. Carbohydrate. Carbohydrates should contribute approximately 50 to 55 percent of the total dietary energy. It is recommended that simple, refined, and other processed sugars provide only about 10 percent of total dietary energy. The remaining carbohydrate calories should come from complex carbohydrates such as starches and naturally occurring sugars found in fruits, vegetables, and milk.

d. Calcium and phosphorus. MRDA are the same for both calcium (Ca) and phosphorus (P), although a wide variation in the Ca:P ratio is tolerated. In the presence of adequate vitamin D nutriture, a ratio of between 1:1 to 1.5:1 is nutritionally desirable.

e. Iron, ascorbic acid, and animal protein. The absorption of iron, a nutrient involved in maintaining optimal aerobic fitness, can be significantly affected by the composition of foods in a particular meal. Heme iron from animal protein sources is better absorbed (approximately 23 percent) than nonheme iron (approximately 3 to 8 percent) which is found in both animal and in many plant food sources. Certain cereal and legume proteins are known to reduce the bioavailability of nonheme iron. The nonheme iron absorption rate can be more than doubled when nonheme iron is consumed with a modest serving of meat, fish, poultry, or a source of ascorbic acid (vitamin C) at the same meal. The dietary iron allowance for females and 17- to 18-year old males is 18 milligrams (mg)/day, or 7.5 and 5.6 mg/1000 calories respectively. Moderately active female personnel consuming an average of 2400 calories per day may require supplemental iron to meet the recommended 18 mg/day. Issuing supplemental iron should be done on an individualized basis after a medical evaluation.

f. Iodine. Wide variation occurs in the amount of iodine present in food and water. All table and cooking salt used should be iodized to ensure an adequate intake of 150 micrograms (mcg) of iodine per day.

g. Fluoride. Fluoride is an essential nutrient which is found in the enamel of teeth and bone. This nutrient is an important factor in preventing tooth decay. Fluoride may confer some protection against certain degenerative bone diseases. Fluoride is found in varying amounts in most foods and water supplies. Maintaining a fluoride concentration of about 1 mg/liter (1 part per million) in water supplies has proven to be safe, economical, and efficient in reducing the incidence of dental caries.

h. Sodium. Sodium is the principal cation involved in maintaining osmotic equilibrium and extracellular fluid volume in the body.

(1) Under conditions of normal ambient temperature and humidity, the healthy adult can maintain sodium balance with an intake of as little as 150 mg/day (381 milligrams of salt). While daily intake below 2000 milligrams of sodium are generally considered upalatable, 3300 milligrams of sodium/day represents a lower acceptable limit to which the American population can adapt. The average young civilian male consumes approximately 5500 milligrams of sodium/day in food plus an additional 20 percent (1000 milligrams) as added salt. Although dietary levels of sodium for the military population are unknown, the average intake may well exceed the civilian level. The goal for the sodium content in foods as served within military dining facilities is 1700 milligrams of sodium/1000 kcal. (See table 3-1.)

(2) Hard physical work in a high ambient temperature greatly increases the amount of sodium lost in sweat. Sodium losses may reach levels as high as 8000 mg/day (20 grams of salt). Whenever more than 3 liters of water per day are required to replace sweat losses, extra salt intake may be required. The need for extra salt depends on the severity of sweat losses and the degree of acclimatization. Sodium should be replaced through food in both nondiscretionary form and as added salt.

i. *Water.* As caloric requirements are increased, water needs are also increased. During periods of light to moderate activity in a temperate climate, 1 milliliter of water per calorie expended is a reasonable intake goal. Water requirements may increase from 50 to 100 percent for personnel living in a hot climate expending similar energy levels. Water requirements may increase threefold above normal under conditions of heavy work in a hot environment. Even in cold climates sweat rates and, consequently, water needs may be quite high due to the hot microclimate that can develop under insulated clothing during heavy physical activity. Inadequate water intakes can be accompanied by a disturbance in electrolyte balance with a resultant performance decrement. (See TB MED 507/NAVMED P-5052-5/AFP 160-1.) Under conditions of normal dietary intake, the preferred fluid to replace losses is cool water. Electrolyte- and sugar-containing solutions are not necessary since glucose and electrolytes are adequately replenished in the normal diet. Under certain conditions, electrolyte and sugar solutions may actually impair rather than enhance performance.

Table 2-1
MRDA for selected nutrients[1]

Nutrient	Unit	Male	Female
Energy[2,3]	Kcal MJ	3200(2800-3600) 13.4(11.7-15.1)	2400(2000-2800 10.0(8.4-11.7)
Protein[4]	gm	100	80
Vitamin A[5]	mcg RE	1000	800
Vitamin D[6,7]	mcg	5-10	5-10
Vitamin E[8]	mg TE	10	8
Ascorbic Acid	mg	60	60
Thiamin (B_1)	mg	1.6	1.2
Riboflavin (B_2)	mg	1.9	1.4
Niacin[9]	mg NE	21	16
Vitamin B_6	mg	2.2	2.0
Folacin	mcg	400	400
Vitamin B_{12}	mcg	3.0	3.0
Calcium[7]	mg	800-1200	800-1200
Phosphorus[7]	mg	800-1200	800-1200
Magnesium[7]	mg	350-400	300
Iron[7]	mg	10-18	18

[1]MRDA for moderately active military personnel, ages 17 to 50 years, are based on the *Recommended Dietary Allowances*, ninth revised edition, 1980.

[2]Energy allowance ranges are estimated to reflect the requirements of 70 percent of the moderately active military population. One megajoule (MJ) equals 239 kcals.

[3]Dietary fat calories should not contribute more than 35 percent of total energy intake.

[4]Protein allowance is vased on an estimated protein requirement of 0.8 gm/kilograms (kg) desirable body weight. Using the reference body weight ranges for males of 60 to 79 kilograms and for females of 46 to 63 kilograms, the protein requirement is approximately 48 to 64 grams for males and 37 to 51 grams for females. These amounts have been approximately doubled to reflect the usual protein consumption levels of Americans and to enhance diet acceptability.

[5]One microgram of retinol equivalent (mcg RE) equals 1 microgram of retinol, or 6 micrograms betacarotene, or 5 international units (IU)

[6]As cholecalcifero, 10 micrograms of cholecalcifero equals 400 IU of vitamin D.

[7]High values reflect greater vitamin D, calcium, phosphorus, magnesium, and iron requirements for 17- to 18-year olds than for older ages.

[8]One milligram of alpha-tocopherol equivalent (mg TE) equals 1 milligram d-alpha-tocopherol.

[9]One milligram of niacin equivalent (mg NE) equals 1 milligram niacin or 60 milligrams dietary tryptophan.

Zinc	mg	15	15
Iodine	mcg	150	150
Sodium	mg	See note[10]	See note[10]

[10]The safe and adequate levels for daily sodium intake of 1100 to 3300 mg published in the RDA are currently impractical and unattainable within military food service systems. However, an average of 1700 milligrams of sodium per 100 kilocalories of food served is the target for military food service systems. This level equates to a daily sodium intake of approximately 5500 milligrams for males and 4100 milligrams for females.

Table 2-2
Estimated safe and adequate daily dietary intake ranges of selected vitamins and minerals[1]

Nutrition	Unit	Amount
Vitamins		
Vitamins K	mcg	70-140
Biotin	mcg	100-200
Pantothenic Acid	mg	4-7
Trace Elements[2]		
Fluoride	mg	1.5-4.0
Selenium	mcg	50-200
Molybdenum	mg	0.15-0.50
Copper	mg	2-3
Manganese	mg	2.5-5.0
Chromium	mcg	50-200
Electrolytes		
Potassium	mg	1875-5625
Chloride	mg	1700-5100

[1]This table is based on the Recommended Dietary Allowances, ninth edition, 1980, table 10, "Estimated Safe and Adequate Daily Dietary Intakes of Selected Vitamins and Minerals." Estimated ranges are provided for these nutrients because sufficient information upon which to set a recommended allowance is not available. Values reflect a range of recommended intake over an extended period of time.

[2]Since toxic levels for many trace elements may only be several times the usual intakes, the upper levels for the trace elements given in this table should not be habitually exceeded.

Table 2-3
Nutritional standards for operational and restricted rations

Nutrient	Unit[1]	Operational rations	Restricted rations[2,4]
Energy	Kcal	3600	1100-1500
Protein	gm	100	50-70
Carbohydrate	gm	440	100-200
Fat	gm	160(maximum)	50-70
Vitamin A	mcg RE	1000	500
Vitamin D	mcg	10	5
Vitamin E	mg TE	10	5
Ascorbic Acid	mg	60	30
Thiamin	mg	1.8	1.0
Riboflavin	mg	2.2	1.2
Niacin	mg NE	24	13
Vitamin B_6	mg	2.2	1.2
Folacin	mcg	400	200
Vitamin B_{12}	mcg	3	1.5
Calcium	mg	800	400
Phosphorus	mg	800	400
Magnesium	mg	800	400
Iron	mg	18	9
Zinc	mg	15	7.5
Sodium	mg	5000-7000[5]	2500-3500[5]
Potassium	mg	1875-5625	950-2800

[1]See notes in table 2-1 for explanation of units.
[2]Values are minimum standards at the time of consumption unless shown as a range or a maximum level.
[3]The operational ration includes the MCI, MRE, A, B, and T rations.
[4]Restricted rations are for use under certain operational scenarios such as long-range patrol, assault, and reconnaissance when troops are required to subsist for short periods (up to 10 days) on an energy restricted ration.
[5]These values do not include salt packets.

C

Dietary Reference Intakes for Calcium and Related Nutrients (IOM, 1997)

FOOD AND NUTRITION BOARD, NATIONAL ACADEMY OF SCIENCES–INSTITUTE OF MEDICINE
DIETARY REFERENCE INTAKES, 1997

	Calcium	Phosphorus		Magnesium		Vitamin D	Fluoride
Life-Stage Group	AI[a] (mg/day)	RDA[b] (mg/day)	AI (mg/day)	RDA (mg/day)	AI (mg/day)	AI[c,d] (μg/day)	AI (mg/day)
Infants							
0 to 6 months	210		100		30	5	0.01
6 to 12 months	270		275		75	5	0.5
Children							
1 through 3 years	500	460		80		5	0.7
4 through 8 years	800	500		130		5	1
Males							
9 through 13 years	1,300	1,250		240		5	2
14 through 18 years	1,300	1,250		410		5	3
19 through 30 years	1,000	700		400		5	4
31 through 50 years	1,000	700		420		5	4
51 through 70 years	1,200	700		420		10	4
> 70 years	1,200	700		420		15	4
Females							
9 through 13 years	1,300	1,250		240		5	2
14 through 18 years	1,300	1,250		360		5	3
19 through 30 years	1,000	700		310		5	3
31 through 50 years	1,000	700		320		5	3
51 through 70 years	1,200	700		320		10	3
> 70 years	1,200	700		320		15	3
Pregnancy							
≤ 18 years	1,300	1,250		400		5	3
19 through 30 years	1,000	700		350		5	3
31 through 50 years	1,000	700		360		5	3
Lactation							
≤ 18 years	1,300	1,250		360		5	3
19 through 30 years	1,000	700		310		5	3
31 through 50 years	1,000	700		320		5	3

[a] AI = Adequate Intake. The observed average or experimentally set intake by a defined population or subgroup that appears to sustain a defined nutritional status, such as growth rate, normal circulating nutrient values, or other functional indicators of health. AI is utilized if sufficient scientific evidence is not available to derive an EAR. For healthy breastfed infants, AI is the mean intake. All other life-stage groups should be covered at the AI value. **The AI is not equivalent to a RDA.**

[b] RDA = Recommended Dietary Allowance. The intake that meets the nutrient need of almost all (97–98 percent) individuals in a group.

[c] As cholecalciferol. 1μg cholecalciferol = 40 IU vitamin D.

[d] In the absence of adequate exposure to sunlight.

FOOD AND NUTRITION BOARD, INSTITUTE OF MEDICINE–NATIONAL ACADEMY OF SCIENCES
DIETARY REFERENCE INTAKES: RECOMMENDED INTAKES FOR INDIVIDUALS

Life-Stage Group	Thiamin (mg/d)	Riboflavin (mg/d)	Niacin (mg/d)[a]	Vitamin B_6 (mg/d)	Folate (µg/d)[b]	Vitamin B_{12} (µg/d)	Pantothenic Acid (mg/d)	Biotin (µg/d)	Choline[c] (mg/d)
Infants									
0–6 mo	0.2*	0.3*	2*	0.1*	65*	0.4*	1.7*	5*	125*
7–12 mo	0.3*	0.4*	4*	0.3*	80*	0.5*	1.8*	6*	150*
Children									
1–3 yr	**0.5**	**0.5**	**6**	**0.5**	**150**	**0.9**	2*	8*	200*
4–8 yr	**0.6**	**0.6**	**8**	**0.6**	**200**	**1.2**	3*	12*	250*
Males									
9–13 yr	**0.9**	**0.9**	**12**	**1.0**	**300**	**1.8**	4*	20*	375*
14–18 yr	**1.2**	**1.3**	**16**	**1.3**	**400**	**2.4**	5*	25*	550*
19–30 yr	**1.2**	**1.3**	**16**	**1.3**	**400**	**2.4**	5*	30*	550*
31–50 yr	**1.2**	**1.3**	**16**	**1.3**	**400**	**2.4**	5*	30*	550*
51–70 yr	**1.2**	**1.3**	**16**	**1.7**	**400**	**2.4**[d]	5*	30*	550*
> 70 yr	**1.2**	**1.3**	**16**	**1.7**	**400**	**2.4**[d]	5*	30*	550*
Females									
9–13 yr	**0.9**	**0.9**	**12**	**1.0**	**300**	**1.8**	4*	20*	375*
14–18 yr	**1.0**	**1.0**	**14**	**1.2**	**400**[e]	**2.4**	5*	25*	400*
19–30 yr	**1.1**	**1.1**	**14**	**1.3**	**400**[e]	**2.4**	5*	30*	425*
31–50 yr	**1.1**	**1.1**	**14**	**1.3**	**400**[e]	**2.4**	5*	30*	425*
51–70 yr	**1.1**	**1.1**	**14**	**1.5**	**400**	**2.4**[d]	5*	30*	425*
> 70 yr	**1.1**	**1.1**	**14**	**1.5**	**400**	**2.4**[d]	5*	30*	425*
Pregnancy									
≤ 18 yr	**1.4**	**1.4**	**18**	**1.9**	**600**[f]	**2.6**	6*	30*	450*
19–30 yr	**1.4**	**1.4**	**18**	**1.9**	**600**[f]	**2.6**	6*	30*	450*
31–50 yr	**1.4**	**1.4**	**18**	**1.9**	**600**[f]	**2.6**	6*	30*	450*
Lactation									
≤ 18 yr	**1.5**	**1.6**	**17**	**2.0**	**500**	**2.8**	7*	35*	550*
19–30 yr	**1.5**	**1.6**	**17**	**2.0**	**500**	**2.8**	7*	35*	550*
31–50 yr	**1.5**	**1.6**	**17**	**2.0**	**500**	**2.8**	7*	35*	550*

NOTE: This table presents Recommended Dietary Allowances (RDAs) in **bold type** and Adequate Intakes (AIs) in ordinary type followed by an asterisk (*). RDAs and AIs may both be used as goals for individual intake. RDAs are set to meet the needs of almost all (97 to 98 percent) individuals in a group. For healthy breastfed infants, the AI is the mean intake. The AI for other life-stage and gender groups is believed to cover needs of all individuals in the group, but lack of data or uncertainty in the data prevent being able to specify with confidence the percentage of individuals covered by this intake.

[a] As niacin equivalents (NE). 1 mg of niacin = 60 mg of tryptophan; 0-6 months = preformed niacin (not NE).

[b] As dietary folate equivalents (DFE). 1 DFE = 1 µg food folate = 0.6 µg of folic acid (from fortified food or supplement) consumed with food = 0.5 µg of synthetic (supplemental) folic acid taken on an empty stomach.

[c] Although AIs have been set for choline, there are few data to assess whether a dietary supply of choline is needed at all stages of the life cycle, and it may be that the choline requirement can be met by endogenous synthesis at some of these stages.

[d] Because 10 to 30 percent of older people may malabsorb food-bound B_{12}, it is advisable for those older than 50 years to meet their RDA mainly by consuming foods fortified with B_{12} or a supplement containing B_{12}.

[e] In view of evidence linking folate intake with neural tube defects in the fetus, it is recommended that all women capable of becoming pregnant consume 400 µg of synthetic folic acid from fortified foods and/or supplements in addition to intake of food folate from a varied diet.

[f] It is assumed that women will continue consuming 400 µg of folic acid until their pregnancy is confirmed and they enter prenatal care, which ordinarily occurs after the end of the periconceptional period—the critical time for formation of the neural tube.

FOOD AND NUTRITION BOARD, NATIONAL ACADEMY OF SCIENCES–NATIONAL RESEARCH COUNCIL RECOMMENDED DIETARY ALLOWANCES,[a] Revised 1989 (Abridged)

Designed for the maintenance of good nutrition of practically all healthy people in the United States

Category	Age (years) or Condition	Weight[b] (kg)	Weight[b] (lb)	Height[b] (cm)	Height[b] (in)	Protein (g)	Vitamin A (μg RE)[c]	Vitamin E (mg α-TE)[d]	Vitamin K (μg)	Vitamin C (mg)	Iron (mg)	Zinc (mg)	Iodine (μg)	Selenium (μg)
Infants	0.0–0.5	6	13	60	24	13	375	3	5	30	6	5	40	10
	0.5–1.0	9	20	71	28	14	375	4	10	35	10	5	50	15
Children	1–3	13	29	90	35	16	400	6	15	40	10	10	70	20
	4–6	20	44	112	44	24	500	7	20	45	10	10	90	20
	7–10	28	62	132	52	28	700	7	30	45	10	10	120	30
Males	11–14	45	99	157	62	45	1,000	10	45	50	12	15	150	40
	15–18	66	145	176	69	59	1,000	10	65	60	12	15	150	50
	19–24	72	160	177	70	58	1,000	10	70	60	10	15	150	70
	25–50	79	174	176	70	63	1,000	10	80	60	10	15	150	70
	51+	77	170	173	68	63	1,000	10	80	60	10	15	150	70
Females	11–14	46	101	157	62	46	800	8	45	50	15	12	150	45
	15–18	55	120	163	64	44	800	8	55	60	15	12	150	50
	19–24	58	128	164	65	46	800	8	60	60	15	12	150	55
	25–50	63	138	163	64	50	800	8	65	60	15	12	150	55
	51+	65	143	160	63	50	800	8	65	60	10	12	150	55
Pregnant						60	800	10	65	70	30	15	175	65
Lactating	1st 6 months					65	1,300	12	65	95	15	19	200	75
	2nd 6 months					62	1,200	11	65	90	15	16	200	75

NOTE: This table does not include nutrients for which Dietary Reference Intakes have recently been established (see *Dietary Reference Intakes for Calcium, Phosphorus, Magnesium, Vitamin D, and Fluoride* [1997] and *Dietary Reference Intakes for Thiamin, Riboflavin, Niacin, Vitamin* B_6*, Folate, Vitamin* B_{12}*, Pantothenic Acid, Biotin, and Choline* [1998]).

[a] The allowances, expressed as average daily intakes over time, are intended to provide for individual variations among most normal persons as they live in the United States under usual environmental stresses. Diets should be based on a variety of common foods in order to provide other nutrients for which human requirements have been less well defined.

[b] Weights and heights of Reference Adults are actual medians for the U.S. population of the designated age, as reported by NHANES II. The median weights and heights of those under 19 years of age were taken from Hamill et al. (1979). The use of these figures does not imply that the height-to-weight ratios are ideal.

[c] Retinol equivalents. 1 retinol equivalent = 1 μg retinol or 6 μg β-carotene.

[d] α-Tocopherol equivalents. 1 mg d-α tocopherol = 1 α-TE.

D

Biographical Sketches

BARBARA O. SCHNEEMAN (Chair) serves as dean, College of Agricultural and Environmental Sciences, and professor of nutrition in the Departments of Nutrition and of Food Science and Technology and in the Division of Clinical Nutrition and Metabolism (School of Medicine), University of California, Davis. Her professional activities include membership on the Dietary Guidelines Advisory Committee, the Board of Trustees of the International Life Sciences Institute America, and editorial boards for *Proceedings of the Society of Experimental Biology and Medicine*, *Food and Nutrition Series* of Academic Press, *Nutrition Reviews*, *Journal of Nutrition*, and *California Agriculture*. Dr. Schneeman's professional honors include the Samuel Cate Prescott award for research, the Future Leader Award, and several honorary lectureships. She received her B.S. in food science and technology from the University of California, Davis; Ph.D. in nutrition from the University of California, Berkeley; and postdoctoral training in gastrointestinal physiology at Children's Hospital in Oakland. Dr. Schneeman's research areas include fat absorption, complex carbohydrates, and gastrointestinal function, and she has a strong interest in and appreciation for nutritional issues that affect women throughout the life cycle.

ROBERT O. NESHEIM (*Vice Chair*) was vice president of Research and Development and later Science and Technology for the Quaker Oats Company until 1983. Before his retirement in 1992, he was vice president of Science and Technology and president of the Advanced Health Care Division of Avadyne, Inc. During World War II, he served as Captain in the U.S. Army. Dr. Nesheim has served on the Institute of Medicine's Food and Nutrition Board, currently chairing the Committee on Military Nutrition Research and formerly chairing the Committee on Food Consumption Patterns and serving as a member of several other committees. He also was active in the Biosciences Information Service (as board chairman), American Medical Association, American Institute of Nutrition, Institute of Food Technologists, and *Food Reviews International* editorial board. Dr. Nesheim's academic services included professor and head of the Department of Animal Science at the University of Illinois, Urbana. He is a fellow of the American Institute of Nutrition and American Association for the Advancement of Science and a member of several professional organizations. Dr. Nesheim holds a B.S. in agriculture, an M.S. in animal science, and a Ph.D. in nutrition and animal science from the University of Illinois.

JOHN P. BILEZIKIAN is presently chief, Division of Endocrinology, and director, Metabolic Bone Diseases Program, Department of Medicine, and professor of medicine and pharmacology, College of Physicians and Surgeons, Columbia University, New York. Dr. Bilezikian received his M.D. from the College of Physicians and Surgeons, Columbia University. He is board certified in internal medicine as well as in endocrinology and metabolism. Most recently, he served as chair for the National Institutes of Health (NIH) Consensus Development Conference on Optimal Calcium Intake and as a member of an NIH special study section on Basic Osteoporosis: New Experimental Strategies (BONES Initiative). He also chaired the Command Osteoporosis Integration Panel for the U.S. Army Medical Research and Materiel Command. He was editor-in-chief for *The Parathyroids: Basic and Clinical Concepts*, associate editor for *Principles and Practice of Endocrinology and Metabolism*, and editor for *Principles of Bone Biology* and has authored over 275 papers on topics of metabolic bone disease and disorders of mineral metabolism.

NANCY F. BUTTE is associate professor of pediatrics, Children's Nutrition Research Center, Department of Pediatrics, Baylor College of Medicine, Houston, Texas. She is a current member of the International Dietary Energy Consultancy Group Steering Committee, Executive Committee for the International Society for Research on Human Milk and Lactation, and Society for International Nutrition Research and a former member of the Institute of Medicine Subcommittee on Nutritional Status and Weight Gain during Pregnancy and of the Expert WHO Committee on Physical Status: The Use and Interpretation of Anthropometry. Dr. Butte received her B.S. in food and nutritional sciences, M.P.H. in public health nutrition, and Ph.D. in nutritional sciences from the University of California, Berkeley, and she is a registered dietitian. Her research experience includes nutritional needs during pregnancy and lactation, including her current focus on military women.

STEVEN B. HEYMSFIELD is professor of medicine at Columbia University, College of Physicians and Surgeons in New York. He also currently serves as deputy director of the New York Obesity Research Center and is director of the Human Body Composition Laboratory. Dr. Heymsfield is immediate past president of the American Society of Parenteral and Enteral Nutrition and is an active member of the American Society of Clinical Nutrition and the North American Society for the Study of Obesity. He was recently made an honorary member of the American Dietetic Association. He received his B.A. in chemistry from Hunter College of the City University of New York and his M.D. from Mt. Sinai School of Medicine. Dr. Heymsfield has done extensive research and has clinical experience in the areas of body composition, weight cycling, nutrition, and obesity, especially as they relate to women.

ANNE LOOKER is senior research epidemiologist, National Center for Health Statistics, Division of Health Examination Statistics, where she serves as the Center's expert consultant on calcium and iron status data for the National Health and Nutrition Examination Surveys. She is currently serving as director of research projects for the National Osteoporosis Foundation and is a member of the National Institute of Arthritis, Musculoskeletal, and Skin Diseases (NIAMS) National Osteoporosis Data Group. Dr. Looker received a B.A. in zoology from Miami University and M.S. and Ph.D. degrees in nutrition from the Pennsylvania State University, and she is a registered dietitian. She has done work in areas that are of special concern to women, such as iron nutrition and osteoporosis.

GORDON O. MATHESON is associate professor and chief of the Division of Sports Medicine at the Stanford University School of Medicine. He is also the director of the Outpatient Sports Medicine clinics at Stanford. Dr. Matheson is heading Stanford's new Academic Sports Medicine program with the development of clinical, research and teaching components. He received his M.D. from the University of Calgary and his Ph.D. in exercise biochemistry from the University of British Columbia. He is a past president of the Canadian Academy of Sport Medicine and is currently the editor-in-chief of the *Clinical Journal of Sport Medicine*. He has served as team physician to the Canadian Olympic Hockey team and the Vancouver Canucks of the National Hockey League and is currently head team physician at Stanford. His research interests include sport and exercise-related injuries and rehabilitation, nuclear magnetic resonance spectroscopy and imaging of skeletal muscle, and hypoxia and altitude acclimatization. He is the author of more than 45 scientific publications.

BONNY L. SPECKER serves as director and chair of the Ethel Austin Martin Endowed Program in Human Nutrition at South Dakota State University. Her professional activities include membership on the Food and Nutrition Board's Panel on Calcium and Related Nutrients and member of several ad hoc National Institutes of Health review panels. She is a member of the Society for Pediatric Research, American Society for Nutritional Sciences, and the American Society for Bone and Mineral Research. She received her B.S. in biology and her Ph.D. in epidemiology from the University of Cincinnati. Dr. Specker's research areas include calcium and vitamin D metabolism in infants and lactating women and the interaction between diet and physical activity on bone mass.

GAIL E. BUTTERFIELD (*CMNR Liaison*) is director of Nutrition Research, Palo Alto Veterans Affairs Health Care System in California. Concurrently, she is lecturer in the Department of Medicine, Stanford University Medical School; visiting assistant professor and co-coordinator of the Health and Human Performance concentration in the Program of Human Biology, Stanford University; and director of nutrition in the Program in Sports Medicine, Stanford University Medical School. Her previous academic appointments were at the University of California, Berkeley. Dr. Butterfield belongs to the American Society for Nutrition Science, American Society for Clinical Nutrition, American Dietetic Association, and American Physiological Society. As a fellow of the American College of Sports Medicine, she serves as chair of the Pronouncements Committee and was recently elected vice president; she also was president and executive director of the Southwest chapter of that organization. She is a member of the Respiratory and Applied Physiology Study Section of the National Institutes of Health and is on the Editorial Boards of the following journals: *Medicine and Science in Sports and Exercise*, *Health and Fitness Journal of ACSM*, *Canadian Journal of Clinical Sports Medicine*, and *International Journal of Sports Nutrition*. Dr.

Butterfield earned her A.B. in biological sciences, M.A. in anatomy, and M.S. and Ph.D. in nutrition from the University of California, Berkeley, and she is a registered dietitian. Her current research interests include nutrition in exercise, effect of growth factors on fuel metabolism in the elderly, and metabolic fuel use at rest and during exercise in women exposed to high altitude.

JANET C. KING (FNB Liaison) is director, U.S. Department of Agriculture Human Nutrition Research Center, Presidio of San Francisco and professor in the Graduate School, University of California, Berkeley. Prior to her university experience, she worked for the U.S. Department of Defense. She is a member of the Institute of Medicine (IOM) and served as chair of the IOM's Food and Nutrition Board and the Subcommittee on Nutrition Status and Weight Gain during Pregnancy. Dr. King received a B.S. in dietetics from Iowa State University and Ph.D. in nutrition from the University of California, Berkeley; she is a registered dietitian.

REBECCA B. COSTELLO (*FNB Staff*) is Project Director for the Committee on Military Nutrition Research and Committee on Body Composition, Nutrition, and Health of Military Women. Prior to joining the FNB staff, she served as Research Associate and Program Director for the Risk Factor Reduction Center, a referral center for the detection, modification and prevention of cardiovascular disease through dietary and/or drug interventions, at the Washington Adventist Hospital in Takoma Park, Maryland. She received her B.S. and M.S. in Biology from the American University, Washington, D.C., and a Ph.D. in clinical nutrition from the University of Maryland at College Park. She has active membership in the American Institute of Nutrition, American College of Nutrition, American Dietetic Association, and American Heart Association Council on Epidemiology. Dr. Costello's areas of research interest include mineral nutrition, dietary intake methodology, and chronic disease epidemiology.

SYDNE J. CARLSON-NEWBERRY (*FNB Staff*) is Program Officer for the Committee on Military Nutrition Research and Committee on Body Composition, Nutrition, and Health of Military Women. Prior to joining the FNB staff, she served as Project Director for the Women's Health Project and Adjunct Assistant Professor in the Department of Family Medicine, Wright State University School of Medicine; as a behavioral health educator for a hospital-based weight management program in Dayton, Ohio; and as a research associate at The Ohio State University Biotechnology Center. She received her B.A. from Brandeis University and her Ph.D. in Nutritional Biochemistry and Metabolism from the Massachusetts Institute of Technology and completed a National Institutes of Health postdoctoral fellowship in the departments of Biochemistry and Molecular Genetics at Ohio State. Dr. Carlson-Newberry's areas of research interest include eating disorders and diabetes management.

E

Abbreviations

AI	Adequate Intake
AIT	Advanced Individual Training
ATP	Adenosine triphosphate
BCNH	Body Composition, Nutrition, and Health of Military Women, Subcommittee
BCT	Basic Combat Training
BMC	Bone Mineral Content
BMD	Bone Mineral Density
BMT	Basic Military Training
BUA	Broadband Ultrasound Attenuation
CI	Confidence Interval
CMNR	Committee on Military Nutrition Research
CR	Cardiorespiratory
CSA	Cross Section Area
CSMI	Moment of Inertia
DEP	Delayed Entry Program
DGGE	Denaturing Gradient Gel Electrophoresis
DHEA	Dehydroepiandrosterone
DoD	Department of Defense

DWHRP	Defense Women's Health Research Project
DXA	Dual X-ray Absorptiometry
EAR	Estimated Average Requirement
FITT	Frequency, Intensity, Time and Type
FSH	Follicle Stimulating Hormone
FTU	Fitness Training Unit
GH	Growth Hormone
GnRH	Gonadotropin Releasing Hormone
HRR	Heart Rate Reserve
IGF-1	Insulin-like Growth Factor-1
IGFBP-1	Insulin-like Growth Factor Binding Protein-1
IL	Interleukin
IOM	Institute of Medicine
LBM	Lean Body Mass
LH	Luteinizing Hormone
MCRD	Marine Corps Recruit Depot
MEPS	Military Entrance Processing Site
MRDA	Military Recommended Dietary Allowance(s)
MRI	Magnetic Resonance Imaging
NPAD	Nonpreganant, Active-duty
NRC	National Research Council
OPHSA	Office of Prevention and Health Services Assessment
OR	Odds Risk
OSUT	One-station Unit Training
NSAID	Nonsteroidal Anti-inflammatory Drug
PC	Physical Conditioning
PCP	Physical Conditioning Platoon
PCR	Polymerase Chain Reaction
PFT	Physical Fitness Test
PGHS-2	Prostaglandin G/H synthase-2
PNF	Proprioceptive Neuromuscular Facilitation
PPFM	Postpartum Family Member
PT	Physical Training
PTH	Parathyroid hormone
PTRP	Physical Training Rehabilitation Program
pDXA	Peripheral Dual X-ray Absorptiometry
pQCT	Peripheral Quantitative Computerized Tomography
QCT	Quantitative Computed Tomography
QTL	Quantitative Trait Localization
QUS	Quantitative Ultrsound
RR	Relative Risk
RTC	Recruit Training Command
SOS	Speed of Sound
SPA	Single Photon Absorptiometry

SSLP	Simple Sequence-length Polymorphism
T3	Triiodothyronine
TGF-β	Transforming Growth Factor-Beta
TNF-α	Tumor Necrosis Factor-alpha
Z	Section Modulus